Acclaim for *Raising the Dead*

"The most beautiful, profound, literary account of what it means to be two beings at once: the traveling soul and the patient rooted to the table, the earth, the body."
—*Los Angeles Times*

"An extraordinary first-person account of retired surgeon Selzer's very close brush with death. . . . This is not a look into the beyond. This is Selzer's personal experience, told in lyric liturgy. Its locale is not beyond, but right on life's border. . . . Whether or not Selzer's narrative is factual, it is a gripping story told with truth."
—*The Philadelphia Inquirer*

"Dramatic and illuminating . . . Selzer helps pull back the veil from our mortality and the intricacies of modern medicine."
—*St. Petersburg Times*

"There is nothing in this clean, simple, superbly reconstructed experience to elicit anything but respect for the considerable talent at work in remembering and bringing courage to others who may someday be in the same boat."
—*The Arizona Daily Star*

"*Raising the Dead* surely will entice anyone curious or interested in life-threatening illness . . . [as] it captures how little we understand about illness, and how wrong it may be to coax the physically and emotionally wounded to move on too fast."
—*Detroit Free Press*

"Told with precision and wit . . . an unsentimental, often funny account of life on the verge of death."
—*Kirkus Reviews*

D0040614

PENGUIN BOOKS

RAISING THE DEAD

Richard Selzer is the author of numerous
books of essays and short stories, including
Down from Troy, *Taking the World in for
Repairs*, and *Mortal Lessons*. His work has
also appeared in many periodicals, among
them *Vanity Fair*, *Harper's*, and *Esquire*. For
many years a professor of surgery at the Yale
School of Medicine, he retired to write full
time. He is the recipient of several honorary
degrees, a National Magazine Award, a
Pushcart Prize for fiction, and a Guggenheim
fellowship. He lives with his wife, Janet, in
New Haven, Connecticut.

Richard Selzer

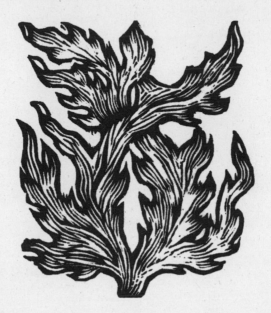

RAISING THE
D·E·A·D

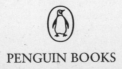

PENGUIN BOOKS

PENGUIN BOOKS

Published by the Penguin Group
Penguin Books USA Inc., 375 Hudson Street,
New York, New York 10014, U.S.A.
Penguin Books Ltd, 27 Wrights Lane, London W8 5TZ, England
Penguin Books Australia Ltd, Ringwood, Victoria, Australia
Penguin Books Canada Ltd, 10 Alcorn Avenue,
Toronto, Ontario, Canada M4V 3B2
Penguin Books (N.Z.) Ltd, 182–190 Wairau Road,
Auckland 10, New Zealand

Penguin Books Ltd, Registered Offices:
Harmondsworth, Middlesex, England

Published in the United States of America by Viking Penguin,
a division of Penguin Books USA Inc., 1994
Published in Penguin Books 1995

1 3 5 7 9 10 8 6 4 2

This book was first published by Whittle Books as part of
The Grand Rounds Press series.
Reprinted by arrangement with Whittle Communications L.P.

LIBRARY OF CONGRESS CATALOGING IN PUBLICATION DATA
Selzer, Richard
Raising the dead/Richard Selzer.
p. cm.
Originally published: Knoxville, Tenn.; Whittle Direct Books, 1993,
in series: Grand rounds press series.
ISBN 0-670-85414-X (hc.)
ISBN 0 14 02.3489 6 (pbk.)
1. Selzer, Richard, 1928—Health. 2. Coma—Patients—United
States—Biography. 3. Legionnaires' disease—Patients—United
States—Biography. 4. Physicians—United States—Biography.
I. Title
RB150.C6S45 1994
362.1´96241—dc20 93–5353
[B]

Printed in the United States of America
Set in Sabon
Designed by Kathryn Parise

for Janet

. . .

In laying myself down like ash after the flame
Have I surrendered?
No, I am sleeping and despite night's power
Learning like a child that I shall awake.

. . .

—PAUL ELUARD

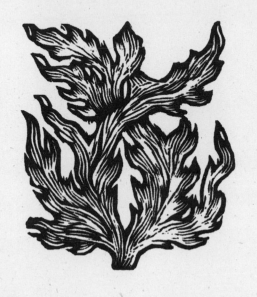

PART ONE

. . .

• • •

It was in August of the year 1810 that Fanny
d'Arblay (née Burney), an Englishwoman living in
Paris and the most famous woman novelist of her
day, experienced for the first time "an annoyance" in
her right breast. Pressing her hand against the discomfort, she felt within its substance a hard lump.
For several minutes she reconnoitered with her fingers, then dismissed the finding from her mind. She
would not think about it. But the pain would not be
dismissed. Within weeks, what had begun as an occasional twinge became a heavy ache from which she
was rarely free. Still, out of fear—some might call it

ignorance—Fanny continued to deny its importance
to herself as well as to her much concerned husband,
Alexandre. Obstinately, she deflected his entreaties to
see a surgeon. Months went by during which the tumor enlarged and the pain intensified. At last,
Fanny's repugnance for a physical examination was
overcome. She would, after all, be examined. It was
Dubois, the most celebrated surgeon of France, who
was summoned—he, because once before she had
been his patient for the successful treatment of an abscess. Dubois looked and palpated and gave the
dreaded news that an operation would be necessary
but that, having recently been appointed *accoucheur*
to the pregnant Empress Josephine, he would not be
free to return until the empress had been safely delivered. Fanny was, by now, distraught. Another name
was suggested, that of Dominique-Jean Larrey, chief
surgeon of the French army and favorite of
Napoleon. Having distinguished himself during the
military campaigns in Egypt, Poland, and Austria,
Larrey had been rewarded with the title of baron by
a grateful commander in chief. It was said that
Larrey had once cured a Polish woman of a similar
malady without surgery.

More terrifying than her pain or the obvious
growth of the tumor was the prospect of an operation, for which Fanny's horror was insuperable. To
be held down, screaming, and cut open like a melon!
Send for Larrey, then, she said at last. But the surgeon proved to be a reluctant consultant, unwilling

to attend her until a letter had been sent by Fanny to
Dubois explaining that her severe fright and continued pain made it impossible to endure the delay oc-
casioned by the royal confinement. Larrey had no
wish to make an enemy of the great Dubois. With the
receipt of that letter and the consent of Dubois, the
case of Fanny d'Arblay was made over to Larrey.

From the first visit, Larrey became the repository
of Fanny's fairest hopes. A nonsurgical regimen was
recommended: compresses, diet, unguents, and rest.
Relief at having escaped the knife and some fortu-
itous lessening of her pain conspired to form Fanny's
opinion that her new doctor was the "most singular-
ly excellent of men, endowed with real Genius in his
profession." Her sharp novelist's eye also took note
of his "ignorance of the world and its usages" and of
a certain naiveté that, to the unfamiliar, might give
him the appearance of being simple and even weak.
"But they would be mistaken," Fanny wrote in her
diary. It is only that "his attention having been
turned exclusively in one way, he is hardly awake in
any other." Over the year of their relationship as
doctor and patient, Fanny and Larrey were to con-
ceive the warmest friendship for each other. This was
to the great benefit of Fanny, who surrendered herself with full trust to his ministrations, but it may
have cost Larrey, who was seduced by his charming
and vivacious patient into stripping off the protective
carapace that is necessary to any man whose work it
is to lay open the bodies of his fellow human beings.

In the weeks that followed, Fanny noted an up-
swing in the level of her energy. With the lessening of
the pain, real or imagined, and no further increase in
the swelling, the lesion had appeared to halt its ad-
vance and even to show signs of subsiding. Although
she still had "cruel seizures," they were shorter and
less frequent. Fanny responded with optimism, declared herself better in every way. She was able to go
out every day and to receive friends at home. Larrey
shared her relief and pronounced himself "enchant-
ed" at her improvement, though apparently not
without some misgivings, as he insisted on another
opinion—that of Ribes, the first anatomist of the na-
tion—lest his own "excessive desire" to spare his patient the agony of surgery had deluded him. To
Fanny's joy, Ribes concurred with Larrey's conserva-
tive treatment.

What, then, was Larrey's consternation when he
returned at the beginning of September 1811, a year
later, to find a marked worsening in the condition of
the breast and a deterioration in the patient's general condition. Not only had the swelling advanced,
but Fanny's right arm had become useless because of
the pain. She required the help of a maid in order to
dress. Why had she not summoned him earlier?

"Et qu'est-il donc arrivé?" he cried. "What is going on here?" The tumor could not be dissolved, he
told her sadly. Surgery would be necessary. Once
again Ribes was called in. Once again he concurred,
corroborating the bad news. Though she could no

longer even climb a flight of stairs without suffering, Fanny, terrified, pleaded for time. A third doctor, the physician Moreau, was summoned. Might he not suggest an alternative? But Larrey had tried everything already. On the day of Moreau's visit, Larrey and Ribes were also present. Together, all three doctors condemned the patient to the operation that she feared more than death itself. With nowhere to turn, Fanny was trapped. Calling up all her reason, if not her courage, she acquiesced. Not all of her anguish could keep her from seeing the tears in the eyes of Larrey. Would she like to be seen by Dubois once more? he offered. Touched by this expression of modesty, Fanny rejected the offer. No, she told Larrey. If she could not be saved by him, she had no hope elsewhere. But now it was Larrey's turn to plead for time. She should obtain the best advice in France, he told her. She was too esteemed, too valued. "The public will be outraged if . . . if . . . you have not the best we can offer you." Perhaps, he said, Dubois might even now suggest a cure without surgery. At that, Fanny was won over. Send for him! Send for him! she cried. But Dubois, fully occupied with his other patients, was not immediately available. He would come as soon as he could, and, furthermore, he would inform her of the date only on that very same day in order to avoid further agitation.

When the time came at last, after a nightmare of waiting, there were four doctors in the salon of the house on the rue de Miromesnil outside of which, with sublime indifference, Paris went on being Paris. Once the examination had been completed, Fanny retired from the room to permit them to consult. After half an hour of torment, she was led back in for the verdict. "All were silent, and Dr. Larrey hid himself nearly behind my sofa. My heart beat fast. I saw all hope was over." It was Dubois himself, disturbed by her plight, who pronounced her doom.

"Will there be much pain?" she asked.

"You must expect to suffer," said Dubois. "I do not wish to fool you. You will suffer greatly."

Now it was the anatomist Ribes who spoke. When the time came, she must not restrain her weeping. To do so would have serious consequences. Hadn't she screamed at the birth of her son? asked Moreau. Yes, she told him. She could not help but do so. Why then, there is nothing to fear, he said. Two things more: Monsieur d'Arblay must not be at home during the time of surgery, and Fanny would not be informed of the date until a few hours ahead. It was the one measure they could take to relieve her anxiety, by shortening its worst period.

And now it was the last day of September, thirteen months since her discovery of the tumor. At 8 A.M. a letter was delivered by a young surgeon, Aumont. In it Larrey wrote that he would arrive at 10 A.M., properly accompanied. He charged her to arrange by whatever subterfuge that her husband be made absent from the house. He exhorted her to rely on his dexterity and experience. Two hours! Larrey again explained that he had deemed it wise to give such short notice to spare her anxiety. With her husband standing by the bedside, Fanny read and reread the letter, her mind darting to think of some ruse by which d'Arblay might be sent away. With all her heart, she wanted to spare this "most loving of men" the sight and sound of her ordeal. Dismissing him momentarily, she sent a note to his employer imploring that an urgent summons call her husband to business and that he be detained until all should be over. That done, Fanny, ever mistress of her household, stifled her fear and told the young surgeon Aumont that she would not be ready until one o'clock. She needed three hours to prepare an apartment for her banished mate; there were nurses to engage, a bed, curtains, heaven knows what, to prepare. Under no circumstances would she be ready until one o'clock. Aumont refused to leave the house and remained in the salon cutting and folding into bandages and sponges the old, fine, castoff underwear he had requested.

At one o'clock, another message came: M. Dubois could not come until three o'clock. Now Fanny, with nothing further to prepare, had only to think and pace. The sight of all those bandages and compresses made her ill. Back and forth, from room to room, she toiled, stilling herself by force of will until she was nearly "torpid."

At last, the clock struck three. There was the clatter of many hooves on the rue de Miromesnil. Fanny raced to the window and saw the cabriolets—one, two, three, four—roll up in quick succession to halt at her door. From each carriage one or two sober-faced men were discharged. With a particular shudder, she recognized Larrey, the man who would, before the hour was up, take up his knife and lay open her body. She retreated to her room. A moment later, the door was opened and seven men in black entered the bedroom of Fanny d'Arblay. It was indignation that roused her from her stupor. Why so many? And without leave! But she could not utter a word of objection.

Once inside, it was Dubois who acted as commander in chief, ordering a bedstead to be placed in the middle of the room, demanding two old mattresses, an old sheet. Fanny was astonished. A bedstead! When Larrey had assured her that an armchair would suffice. She turned to him for confirmation but Larrey kept himself out of sight, at the periphery of the hubbub, his head downcast, his eyes averted. Fanny felt herself trembling, losing control of her nerves. The operating theater having been arranged to his satisfaction, Dubois bid her mount the bedstead. For a moment, she had an impulse to race to the door, the window, and escape. But reason reinstated itself and she stood her ground.

"Please remove your robe," said Dubois, issuing the command *en militaire*. Her robe! She had meant

to keep it on. But submit she did. Oh how she longed
for her sisters, all so far away, or a friend who would
protect her modesty. At the evidence of her despair
Dubois softened and spoke a few soothing words.
But Fanny did not hear.

"Can you," she cried out to him, "can you imagine how I approach this operation that, *to you*, must
seem so trivial?"

"Trivial?" he repeated, and in his discomfort he
took up a bit of paper and tore it unconsciously into
pieces. *"Oui,"* he stammered, "it is a small thing . . .
but . . . ," and could not go on. Somehow Dubois'
agitation canceled her defensiveness. A glance at
Larrey, who remained at the farthest reaches of the
room, showed her a face as pale as ashes. Then
Fanny knew the enormity of her danger. Unbidden
now, she mounted the bedstead. Dubois settled her
upon the mattress and spread a cambric handkerchief over her face—a pitiful blindfold through
which she could see that the bed was surrounded by
the seven men. Hands were laid upon her, to hold.
Through the cambric she saw the glitter of polished
steel, then closed her eyes and waited. A long silence
ensued in which she imagined that the surgeons dis-
coursed with signs. At last someone spoke.

"Who will hold the breast?" It was the solemn,
melancholy voice of Larrey. No one answered.
Through the handkerchief, she saw the hand of
Larrey above her breast describing with his finger the

lines of his incision. A straight line from top to bottom, a cross, and a circle, intimating that the whole breast was to be taken off.

Unable to keep still any longer, Fanny started up, threw off her veil, cupping her breast from the bottom to present it to the surgeons, she cried: "Who will hold the breast? *C'est moi, Monsieur*. I will." Swiftly and firmly Dubois replaced her as before, covering her face again with the handkerchief. Fanny closed her eyes, and waited. It was the moment of incision.

When it came, she felt the knife drawn about her breast followed by a wake of pain "like a mass of forked poniards tearing." Fanny needed no encouragement to let herself go, but heard from her own throat an animal howl such as she had not thought a human capable of, a howled vowel that was interrupted only by the need for more breath to propagate itself anew. She imagined the knife describing a curve, now cutting against the grain as the resistant flesh opposed and tired the hand of the surgeon who must again and again change the knife from one hand to the other. At last the knife withdrew. *It is over*, she thought. But no. In the next moment, the thing lowered its snout to feed again, more voraciously than ever, as it separated the "dreadful gland" from the parts to which it was adherent.

"*Ah, messieurs*," she cried. "*Que je vous plains!* How sorry I am for you!" Again a pause as Larrey rested his hand. Again the scalpel lowered, now audibly raking against her breastbone. Scraping! At last, in the midst of her agony, Fanny felt that the knife had been withdrawn from her flesh. There was a pause, after which she heard Larrey ask his colleagues "in a tone nearly tragic" if anyone saw a need to cut away any more tissue.

"Yes," came the voice of Dubois, and she could *feel* his finger pointing above the wound. The cutting resumed. Another pause. Now Moreau discerned another peccant atom. Again Dubois, demanding yet a bit more flesh. And another. Just before losing consciousness, the screaming woman cried out: "In the name of God, what are you doing to me?"

Her next memory was of being lifted and carried to her own bed. Only then did she open her eyes to see Larrey looking down at her, "pale nearly as myself, his face streaked with blood, and its expression depicting grief, apprehension and almost horror." The operation, from incision to closure, had taken twenty minutes. To Fanny it had seemed twenty years. In this account, given by Fanny nine months later in a letter to her sister, the dramatic terms in which the event is rendered are those of the novelist whose heroine is not unlike Joan of Arc. Hadn't Fanny mounted her bedstead as bravely as Joan of Arc her stake? Hadn't she "forgiven" her surgeons much as Joan had forgiven the men who convicted her? Hadn't Cardinal Beaufort and the judges wept as they sealed the fate of the Maid of Orléans even as the surgeon Larrey's eyes had filled with tears? Her utterances themselves are those of a martyr. If no one else, then she, Fanny, would present her breast to the knife. "How sorry I am for you," she had cried. Only in her last outcry: "What are you doing to me?" is there any human spontaneity. As for the rest, they are the words of the supremely self-conscious and melodramatic novelist. One hastens to forgive her entirely for her self-indulgence.

In the postoperative report, written the next day by one of Larrey's pupils, we read:

At 3:45 on September 31, 1811, Mme. d'Arblay submitted to the removal of a fist-sized cancer that originated in the right breast and was adherent to the pectoralis major muscle. The operation was performed by M. le baron Larrey, assisted by Professor Dubois and Drs. Moreau, Ribes, and Aumont. It was very painful and endured with great courage. The center of the tumor showed early cancerous degeneration, but all its roots were excised, and in no other case has so serious an operation promised more hope of success.

The extreme sensibility of the patient caused the most violent postoperative spasms which were only controlled by the use of sedatives. The patient had an uncomfortable night—full of agitation, spasms, headaches, nausea, and vomiting. . . . But by ten in the morning the patient was astonished to find herself alive and fairly comfortable. Upon his arrival, M. Larrey found her to be without fever, and with very little pain and virtually no bloody drainage. . . .

He prescribed cream of rice soup and a jelly of
meat. Also, chicken soup and a decoction of
thickened barley water with lemon. This evening
she took a second decoction of linseed and the
flower heads of the poppy.

Although nothing in the scanty report indicates
the nature of the incision, the type of sutures, or the
measures used to control bleeding, it is possible to in-
fer what took place from what is known of Larrey's
technique as it is described in his *Memoirs of
Military Surgery*. The incision may be assumed to
have been of the simple guillotine, or circular, type,
as was used in the performance of so many amputa-
tions on the battlefield. Surely, this would have been
the quickest way to remove the breast. In the absence
of anesthesia and in the desire to cause as little bleeding and surgical shock as possible, speed was essen-
tial. Larrey was known to have amputated a
shattered arm or leg in three minutes from the incision in the skin to its closure without sutures. In any
operation, only the largest of the blood vessels were
ligated with waxed cotton thread, the rest being allowed to stop of their own accord by clotting, or by
use of cautery with a hot iron. To close the wound,
flaps of skin with its underlying fat would have been
undercut, loosened, and lifted to meet similar flaps
from the opposite margin. The edges of apposed skin
would then have been sutured. But loosely, with gaps
left between the stitches to allow for egress of blood,

serum, and any tissue injured or destroyed during the procedure, and above all, to allow for the release of pus. To Larrey, as to all other surgeons of his time, the sight of pus streaming from a wound forty-eight hours after surgery was cause to rejoice, as it meant that in all likelihood, the underlying tissues were healing. Pus to these surgeons was "laudable." They gave thanks for it. Suppuration having been established, one had only to wait for new tissue to build up from the base of the wound and for the skin to grow across the separated edges. Any more meticulous approximation of the wound would surely serve to seal in the inevitable pus and invite complete breakdown of the wound or worse: blood poisoning and death.

The diagnosis was cancer of the breast. From the beginning Fanny had experienced pain, heaviness, and tenderness. Within months the function of her arm had become impaired so as to keep her from dressing herself or writing. In time, she could not climb a flight of stairs without exhaustion. The mass was visibly and palpably enlarging. At the time of the surgery, it had reached the size of a man's fist. Moreover, it was noted to have extended into the muscles of the chest. What else could it be but a cancer?

It is not to take away from Larrey's singular achievement—only twice before, in 1655 and again in 1718, had mastectomy been performed for what was thought to be cancer of the breast—nor to demythologize Fanny's novelistic account of her peril that one must, in retrospect, have some reason to doubt the accuracy of the diagnosis. Fanny d'Arblay lived for twenty-nine years after her operation, surviving both her husband and her son. It is unlikely that so locally extensive a cancer would have been eradicated by an operation that did not include removal of the lymph nodes under the arm. Although such a large and longstanding cancer might have remained confined, it is more apt to have broken out of its bounds and spread via the bloodstream or the lymphatic ducts to distant parts of the body.

What else might it have been? A chronic, indolent abscess—syphilitic, tubercular, or otherwise bacterial—can by compression of the adjacent tissues produce about itself a hard, fibrous capsule that would give the mass the feel of a solid tumor when in fact it is a cavity containing liquid or semisolid material, such as is described in the operative report. Such an abscess would excite in the surrounding tissues an inflammation which would cause the lesion to adhere to the underlying chest wall so as to give the impression of tumor extension when it might have been no more than inflammatory tissue. A chronic abscess of this type could produce infected lymph glands in the armpit and so give rise to pain in the arm itself. Against such a diagnosis is the great age of the lesion, at least thirteen months. By then, an abscess could be expected to have produced redness and swelling of the skin. The natural course of such a lesion is to grow ever more superficial until at last it bursts forth to the outside.

Another, more likely diagnosis is cystosarcoma phyllodes, a usually benign tumor that can grow to great size before stabilizing. It is not unheard of for such a tumor to grow so quickly that it outstrips its own blood supply and undergoes necrotic degeneration at its core. Here too, the inflammatory response could produce adherence to the chest wall. The pain in Fanny's arm could have been referred from the breast via the branches of the brachial plexus of nerves in the armpit. Against this diagnosis is Fanny's age, fifty-nine, far older than most, but not all, women who develop this benign tumor.

Fanny d'Arblay had been a literary lioness, admired by Samuel Johnson, Edmund Burke, Thomas Macaulay, and Jane Austen (who took the title of her book *Pride and Prejudice* from Fanny's novel *Cecilia*) for over a quarter of a century, since the publication of her first novel—*Evelina*, the story of a young girl's entry into English society—in 1778. Each of her novels was awaited as impatiently as those of Sir Walter Scott. Throughout her life she moved in brilliant aristocratic circles both in her native England and in Paris, where she lived with her French husband, Count Alexandre d'Arblay. It was enough to turn any writer's head. And it did.

From her voluminous diary, it is not hard to form the portrait of a vain, opinionated woman with an insatiable appetite for compliments, yet vivacious, witty, effusive to the point of hysteria, shallow but never insincere, and with an immense gift for friendship. And with a novelist's eye for detail. In her own eyes, she was saintly, just, affectionate, and too often victimized by the less high-souled and the jealous. To the historian striving for impartiality, she emerges as a difficult but fascinating woman with a kind of full-dress elegance, understandably adored by her less flamboyant husband and son, about whom she orbited like a luminous moon. A woman who grew, not up, only older.

How far from the unvarnished facts the novelist strayed in the recapitulation of her martyrdom one cannot, and would not, say. Such ignoble doubting is for the cynics of medicine and literature, of whom there is no lack. The only account was written in a letter to her sister nine months after her surgery. How far, after all, from the facts of the Passion of Jesus Christ are the much delayed writings of Matthew, Mark, Luke, and John, each of which differs significantly from the others? Besides, what writer has not overshot a mark or two in his time? History is as much a matter of opinion as it is of fact. Whatever else is open to question in the case of Fanny d'Arblay, her suffering is most emphatically authentic. What happened, happened. A woman had a tumor of the breast. A surgeon removed it without anesthesia. The woman was cured.

And what of the surgeon Larrey? With tears in

his eyes and a face "pale as ashes" at the thought of
the suffering of his patient? Could this be the first
surgeon of the French army who at age forty-five had
already accompanied Napoleon on his campaigns to
Egypt and Syria, Austria, Poland, and Spain? Who
had, with legendary courage, performed thousands
of operations on the field of battle amid showers of
bullets and whirlwinds of snow and sand, often with
no more shelter than a cloak held over the patient by
two men during the procedure?

Of a surgeon it is said that he is but an extension
of his scalpel, a man whose emotions must be held
prisoner in the deepest compartment of the heart lest
he be unmanned and his resolve fail him. As this is
not true of the majority of surgeons (women, now, as
well as men), it was not true of Larrey. So unblunted
was he, even in the midst of the calamities of war,
that he was unable to refrain from tears at the
screams of the wounded and the misery of the
soldiers which it was not in his power to alle-
viate. Possessed of genius himself, Larrey worshiped
genius in others, whether it resided in a famous
woman writer or in Napoleon Bonaparte, whose
exile on Elba he was only deterred from sharing by
Napoleon's insistence that he remain with the army
of France.

Months later, in the new intimacy between Fanny
and Larrey born out of the shared experience of
having gazed together into the mouth of hell, Larrey
was to reveal to Fanny d'Arblay that he too had all

had all but lost his nerve. It seems that at the time of the last consultation, Dubois had declared the lesion inoperable, the cancer too far advanced for surgical removal. Any operation could only hasten her death. At that moment, Larrey, in the words of Fanny, "regretted to his soul ever having known me, and was on the point of demanding a commission to the furthest end of France in order to force me into other hands." Hyperbole? Perhaps, but entirely forgivable in the convalescent's portrayal of her ordeal and rescue. It is a small pleasure considering the suffering that went before. It is a pleasure of which few patients hesitate to avail themselves. "Mine," a visitor is told, "was the largest kidney stone my doctor had ever seen." That sort of thing.

Larrey died at the age of seventy-two, two years after the death of Fanny d'Arblay. It is one of those ironic judgments of history that Larrey, the surgeon, was to outlive Fanny, the novelist, in the matter of literary reputation as well.

With the arguable exception of her first novel, *Evelina*, the rest of her literary output, hugely popular in its day, has not stood the test of time. It is undistinguished, some say unreadable, and justly forgotten. Whereas the military and surgical memoirs of Baron Larrey are masterpieces of medical history, rendered in prose so meticulous and sharp as to suggest having been written with something other than a pen. A scalpel, perhaps? Here he is on the treatment of frostbite during the campaign in Russia:

It will easily be conceived why, instead of submitting the part to heat which provokes gangrene, it is necessary to rub the affected part with substances containing very little calorie. Snow and ice are the substances to which recourse should be had. Should this fail, the part ought to be plunged in cold water until bubbles of air are seen to disengage themselves from the congealed part. This is the process adopted by the Russians for thawing a fish. If they soak it in warm water, they know from experience that it will become putrid in a few minutes; whereas, after immersion in cold water, it is as fresh as if it had just been caught.

Now show me the writer who wouldn't die to have written that.

• • •

IN 1624, the poet John Donne, vicar of Saint Dunstan-in-the-West, took to his bed with a grave illness that brought him to the verge of death. A precise diagnosis was never made, although the disease was characterized by fever, rash, and cough. Most likely were two possibilities: typhus and so-called relapsing fever, both of which have been indicted as the cause of the epidemic fever that swept London in 1623 and 1624. The acute illness lasted about three weeks, presumably the length of time needed for the disease to burn itself out. Donne himself survived and went on to contract tuberculosis two years later, and cancer of the stomach some six years after that. During the acute illness, Donne jotted down notes that described his spiritual reactions to his physical state. These later formed the basis of his *Devotions Upon Emergent Occasions*, twenty-three sets of prose pieces, each consisting of a prayer, an expostulation, and a meditation. Taken all together they constitute a spiritual quest inspired by a dangerous illness. In writing of her illness, Fanny d'Arblay was the consummate storyteller making the literary most of what happened to her; in writing of his, John Donne was the philosophic divine, seeking the meaning of affliction.

Now it would seem only natural that a convalescent scrivener, having survived his own dangerous illness, should attempt to follow in the footsteps of two such eminent writers. But I did not share Madame d'Arblay's charming yen to make romance out of life. And long years of skepticism have distanced me from prayer and expostulation, both of which imply a presence that will respond. That leaves meditation, the only category that needs no one but the narrator himself. And so I shall begin to meditate.

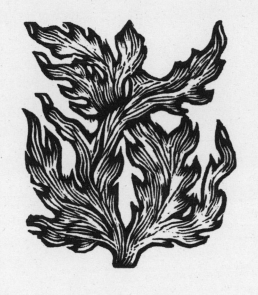

PART TWO

. . .

. . .

On the evening of March 31, 1991, in a house on St. Ronan Terrace, I sat writing in the room I call my scriptorium. Usually, in Connecticut March is winter hanging by a thread, but this year it had turned hot without any transitional period of moderation; the leaves were already half-size. For most of the month I had been on an extended lecture tour that took me from the island of Kauai to Nova Scotia, then on to Delaware, California, and Texas. Around nine o'clock I left my desk and went to stand at the open window. The branches had begun to stir in a sudden breeze. There was the muffled sound of thunder.

Jagged nerves of lightning leaped. In the sultry air the pattern of the wallpaper turned from green to gold; the figures in it grew wavy, they vibrated like heat rising from a pavement. All at once, my legs buckled. From downstairs Janet heard the thud and came running.

"What?" she said.

"I can't think why . . . ," I replied.

"Can you get up?" I tried but could not.

"You'd better call . . ." But she had already dialed. Within minutes two young men in uniform stood over me. I remember being bundled up, the stretcher sliding home aboard the ambulance. One of the men took my pulse and blood pressure, then relayed the information to someone over the phone. I heard the sirens.

"For goodness' sake, don't use the sirens," I told him. "It will disturb the neighbors. Besides, it isn't that serious."

"Take it easy, Pops," said the young man. "It's sporty this way." I remember nothing else until twenty-three days later when I woke up on a ship, I thought; somewhere off the coast of Texas, I thought. Oh yes, there was this: at the emergency room I was placed on a stretcher. All around and above me, a flock of white birds—stooping to peck at my arms, groins, beaking my mouth, rectum, everywhere. Then nothing . . . save for whispers crowding around, leading me deeper and deeper into the darkness. Then they too vanished.

Coma is the state into which he is tumbling. Moment by moment, there is a turning inward of the senses. The sounds, smells, sights, perceptions of the outside world are disappearing. The Milky Way roars across the sky like an army of light. At last, his fall is broken by a soft cushion and he is suspended in a viscous, pearly matrix that is itself both time and space; his vertebrae have melted; he lies here strewn, submerged.

I feel ashamed to pounce upon the page with a narrative that is so open, explicit, so personal. In one sense it is a vivisection, the cutting up of a living creature to see how it works, rummaging among the still-quivering flesh for its soul. As you can see, I am warming up before making a start, rubbing my hands together to summon up courage. If I have written much of it in the third person, well, that is because such an obsessive account of an illness forces one, like Dorian Gray, to confront his own "devilish, furtive, ingrown" self-portrait. The pronoun *he* gives a blessed bit of distance between myself and a too fresh ordeal in which the use of *I* would be rather like picking off a scab only to find that the wound had not completely healed. Still, *I*, the author, will be present throughout, looking on, translating for *him*, the patient.

In writing this journal, I had no overriding wish to educate myself in the subject of Legionnaires' disease, the diagnosis ultimately given to my ailment. Once I had learned that it is caused by the bacterium

Legionella pneumophila, which thrives in the mist sprayed from air-conditioning ducts, that a building or an airplane having been infested, travelers are especially vulnerable, that it is quite often a massive pneumonia associated with collapse of the respiratory function and therefore fatal; once I had glanced at a few colored photographs of autopsy specimens of lungs and liver and kidney, my curiosity about the disease was exhausted. A writer, like an old-time doctor, prefers impressions to facts. Impressions are what last. Facts, such as the data read from the screen of the computer, have a tendency to change from day to day. But I think it is time to get on with the chronicle of an illness told afterward.

Let us look in upon that cubicle of the emergency room. The stretcher upon which he lies is engulfed in nurses and doctors, each of whom is ministering to him at the same time. In a moment, his clothing is stripped from him. Because he is flailing about, his wrists and ankles have been restrained. From veins in his arms and groins endless ribbons of blood, dark from the cyanosis, are pulled into tubes. His head is steadied, his neck extended by mighty hands; the mouth of the man is pried open and an attempt is made to insert a tube into his trachea. But his agitation is extreme, like that of a man drowning. Or rather, that of a man playing the role of someone drowning in an old-fashioned melodrama. It has that jerky, staccato rhythm. Because of this, the intubation cannot be carried out. Medication is injected

into a vein and the doctor at the head of the stretcher tries again.

There. Now the tube is in his trachea, the cuff inflated to keep it from slipping out. Still not fully nar-
cotized, the man shakes his frantic head from side to
side, refusing what has been thrust in. He coughs,
strains, his neck is a contraption of taut tendons and
engorged veins. To the uninitiated it might seem a
kind of molestation. At last the morphine reaches his
brain; he subsides into flaccidity. His chest lifts, re-
cedes, lifts again at the insistence of the rhythmic,
squeezing fist of a perfect stranger. Ointment is
squeezed from a tube into his eyes, and his lids are
taped shut to protect the corneas. It is the beginning
of a long sleep. In the meantime, a catheter has been
slid into his bladder, another plastic tube into one of
his nostrils to gain access to his stomach. Already,
long strings of blackish bile are staining the sheet on
which he lies. The cardiogram shows the rhythm of
his heart to be precarious—ventricular tachycardia.
Drugs are administered, electrodes readied to apply
to the chest. An X-ray is taken; one of the doctors re-
marks that the chest is not expanding symmetrically.
The diagnosis is massive bilateral pneumonia with
toxic shock. How strange that he had no earlier
warning. Despite the administration of pure oxygen,
his lips and fingernails remain blue. His temperature,
they say, is very high. His pulse too, his blood pressure almost obtainable. Is he going to die? No one
knows. But there is more than a hint of death here.

Within minutes, then, he is a preparation, something they have made and whose every flicker and seepage can be measured precisely. In addition to the doctors, nurses and technicians, I, the author, am also there standing, or rather, hovering bodiless above and to the side, out of the way yet able to see, to hear, now and then able to reach down if I wish and touch him, the one lying there on the stretcher who seems to me a small bird perched on an arrow that has been shot from the bow and is flying somewhere. If ever the man wakes up and can speak for himself, I shall have to change pronouns.

The martyrdom of the intensive care unit has begun. It has a certain relentless monotony which would render any such narrative boring. So I shall not proceed day by day through the pestering and goading of the flesh that go by the name intensive care. Suffice it to say that for the next twenty-three days the man in the bed is to be ventilated, dosed, defibrillated, probed, suctioned, and infused. Most of his bodily functions will be taken over. No longer need he swallow, chew, inhale or exhale, cough, urinate, defecate, clear his throat, maintain acid-base balance, cogitate, remember, sigh, weep, laugh, desire. Even the need for making tears has been taken over by the ophthalmic ointment that protects his corneas. For those who will tend him, he is at once the raison d'être and the predicament from which they long to extricate themselves. The doctors are earnest and tireless. They remind me of poor farmers who, year in and year out, turn with their hoes the same exhausted patch of soil, planting and replanting, flogging it, cherishing it. But there will come the day when the pathetic patch of dust will no longer yield. Only then will they let it be. In other words, this man is half-dead, although not quite at the point of no return. For him death would certainly be much easier to achieve than life. The prospect of life regained is like sitting down to a gourmet lunch without the blessing of appetite.

The intensive care unit suggests a blockhouse, a building made of concrete, designed to withstand attack during wartime. Even the patient who is conscious exists here in a kind of reverie. Within the blockhouse twenty respirators, each inhaling at its own pace, make a steady, wet noise like the fall from a fountain. Such a sound goes unnoticed in an intensive care unit beneath the clatter and thump, the footfalls, the calling out, the moaning. So cleverly has the noise of these respirators been woven into the larger fabric of sound that within minutes it cannot be dissected and analyzed for itself. Absolute silence could not be deeper. All the while, in the chimney of his brain, thoughts fly up and, a moment later, waft away, irretrievable.

Dreamer that he is, even in the blockhouse, even from the depths of his coma, he invites the IV pole, the respirator, the whole massive bank of machinery to suggest the background for a story: the hanging bottles of saline become a crystal chandelier; the

moans of his sick neighbor are the sound of an oboe
being played in another part of the house; the cooing
of pigeons on the window ledge becomes the rapturous cries of lovers. Those who enter and leave his
room will be characters in a story—there is a nurse,
Maureen, with a long, slender neck at the hollow of
which rests a tiny gold cross. A chambermaid per-
forms her futile acts of domesticity, fitting her mop in
and around the legs of the others. Now and then, she
will cast a glance at the wreckage in the bed and sigh.
Even to death and beyond, he will be the teller of
tales, collecting impressions, defying forgetfulness,
and meeting gods all along the road, the way you do
when reading Homer or Virgil. He can do all that? In
coma? Oh yes, he can. Dream, imagination—these
are the chariots that the comatose body rides. It is by
these that the flesh extends itself to encompass the
whole world.

He had always been thin—a parcel of bones really, stitched together with ligament, strung with
nerves and tendons, and with a cap of aluminum
hair; his eyes are of that indeterminate color called
hazel. But now it is the sixth day. He is swollen like a
toad, his flesh cold and soggy, his edematous eyelids
at half-mast. You wonder how they could have over-
hydrated him so. In their zeal to combat his state of
shock, they have given him fifty pounds of excess
glucose and saline solution. There is the sadness of a
toad in his hazel eyes. The familiar landmarks by
which he could once be identified are no longer to be

seen: the zygomatic arches surmounting the cheeks, the iliac crests, the tapered phalanges. Where is the squarish mandible that (he has been told) gave his head the look of a Roman senator? Where, the graceful hollow above each clavicle? And all the while, beneath the deceptive fullness of edema, the wasting of his muscles goes on, the congestion of his internal organs. He has become something that even I would not want to touch. Not so the nurses—Maureen, Linda, Heather. Beautifully serene, they continue to stroke and massage him, to wipe away all stains, to bathe and dress him in clean linen. To look at him today you would never guess that he is the same man brought to the emergency room six days ago and set loose at supersonic speed into the void and traveling on remote control.

· · ·

AT LAST, by the tenth day, the diuretic has succeeded in drying him out. Succeeded beyond anyone's expectations. All day and all night, the nurses have emptied the plastic collecting bags suspended from the siderail of the bed, exclaiming. The output of urine is nothing short of heroic. Within four days he has become little more than a skeleton, every bone visible and palpable—the skeleton of a child whose puberty has been delayed. At the same time, he looks ancient enough to have been mentioned in the Old Testament. Oh, let me confess it! Sometimes he seems brave and beautiful to me, although I know that I am the only one who would think so. Look at him! A sprig of chicory blooming between paving stones, indomitable.

Day Fourteen. All the blood that is still in a liquid state has been drawn from his veins; syringe after syringe has glittered with it. The rest is clotted or extravasated into the tissues. Huge purpura, ecchymoses, and hematomas cover the sticks that were his arms. There is a moist rattle in the endotracheal tube. Now and then, a nurse detaches the tube from the respirator long enough to suction it clear, and then the rattle disappears for a while.

I have spent the entire day observing him. The poverty of his body, the way he shivers like a wet dog. The draining away of his flesh and blood. He is like an abandoned cottage in ruins, the eaves of his ribs overhanging the scaphoid belly. His umbilicus, that mute evidence of his ancestry, seems set directly upon the vertebral column. When the narcosis is allowed to lift, he curls up, stretches out slowly like a larva, signaling with the only sound he can make— the faint borborygmi of his bowel. At last I understanding the term *embedded*, the way a fly trapped in a chunk of amber must apprehend its plight.

Beneath the sheet he is naked save for his feet, which are encased in brand-new high-top running shoes. His wife has shopped for them at the suggestion of Maureen, who is worried about foot drop.

These massive sneakers hold the feet at right angles to the legs. It is ludicrous, and even the anguished members of his family—his children—cannot keep from smiling at the small boy who has taken his new shoes to bed with him.

Day Eighteen. He has been in coma for almost three weeks. What is it like? It is like being encased in a layer of wax that separates him from the rest of mankind. The outer air is a foreign element into which he is unable to break through. Nor should he try, for he could no longer breathe it in. An immense weight holds down his thin bluish eyelids. He could not have raised them. Nor does he want to. He has no need for eyes. Here, there is nothing for him to do but wait and listen to the silences rubbing against each other. Now and then there is a small shifting in the air as if far away, on another continent, a boa constrictor were slowly unwinding from a branch. Could this place have a name? Is it on any map of the world? A decision has been made to wean him from the respirator.

The narcotics and paralyzing agents have been given in lower doses throughout the night. Toward dawn he is lying in the upper berth of a sleeping car; there is no room to sit up or turn over. The train is hurtling across an endless prairie where it is always night. Once in a while the eternal darkness outside the train window is punctuated by something—a forest of bare white birch trees, a herd of cattle, only their white faces showing. A few silvery birds fly. Or are they fish streaming?

There are times when his face seems to contort into weeping; his eyes open and show themselves brimming with a molten sorrow. When it passes, the spasm, there is a relief about the diaphragm as when vomiting or sobbing stops and you can let go of yourself. This morning he even made a gesture as if to reach up and claw from him the skin of wax that is his coma. It is the same gesture made by Lazarus in the painting (School of Rembrandt) when he sits up in the tomb and begins to unwrap his cerements. But unlike Lazarus, the man in bed cannot manage it. By afternoon his arms and legs are once again flailing about, resisting. In the chart his behavior is noted as "combative." Nothing could be further from the truth. What makes him struggle so is not aggressiveness; it is desperation.

The man now is about the size of a small deer lying starved and exhausted in snow. See how he lifts his head, turns it slowly, on his face a look of puzzlement, uncertainty, as he sees me hovering in the corner of the room where wall and ceiling meet. Something passes between us—not quite speech. He opens his mouth as if to eject the tube but cannot. Then with a purposefulness that I did not think he could muster, he reaches one hand up and pulls it, coughing, choking, from his throat with the cuff still inflated. He seems surprised at what he has done, the sounds he is making.

"That was very naughty!" The nurse attaches nasal prongs to deliver oxygen to his nostrils until the doctor can come to replace the tube. Meanwhile, he is rid of the tube and struggles to extrude vowels and consonants from his larynx. Even his eyebrows take part in the effort to speak, the way they arch, lifting as if to encourage his lips and tongue. It gives his face a look of boyish earnestness. But there is no voice, only a thick, gelatinous rasp, as the vocal cords no longer approximate. Minutes later, the anesthesiologist arrives. Just in time, for the cyanosis has darkened. The wrists and ankles of the patient have been secured to the bed. The nurse holds his head as if it were the head of a statue whose sightless eyes have no pupils. The hands that grip him are hard as tongs. In the end he yields to them as though yielding to a strangler's thumbs. The endotracheal tube is replaced, its cuff inflated. The dose of morphine is increased. Immediately, his empty sockets return a gray, stony stare. He must remain paralyzed and unconscious until such time as he no longer needs the respirator. And so he sleeps on.

· · ·

HE IS LIKE a gardener digging in the earth who makes a decision to lower himself to the underworld. Down and down he goes, swinging from root to root. On either side, worms, rocks, gulches, darkness, eyes like panthers caught in a net of lashes, moisture dripping. Just so does he follow the mushroom scent of hell, and with each fathom grows paler, less opaque, his flesh melting—solid to liquid, until at last there will be only the vagueness of vapor. Once or twice he looks back up to see how far he has come, but the path behind has closed up, leaving no trace. He would not be able to find his way back. The thick, twisted roots have tapered into fine, hairlike rhizomes that he parts with his hand the way one parts a curtain of beads. His cheeks and arms are coated with cold moisture, more like rot than sweat. The odor of mushrooms grows heavier. Solid ropes of it slide in and out of his mouth, fill his throat. After a long time, the path widens and ends abruptly at the edge of a black river. Here he lies down, not to sleep—in this place there is no need for sleep or wakefulness. Nor is there any need to move.

Day Twenty. The sight of his hands is particularly sad. Those fine muscles between the metacarpal bones and in the web spaces—the interossei and the lumbricals—have atrophied; the mounds of flesh have given way to gullies. The skin is dry and as chaste and beautiful as old paper. But I remember the passion inspired by those fingers, their gifted, sly, infinitely provocative caresses and gestures. No sign of that now.

A doctor turns over first one hand, then the other,

searching perhaps for a usable vein. Then he sees the elevated, dimpled scar tissue in each palm that begins to contract and draw down the ring finger. That is the Dupuytren's contracture of which the man has been inordinately proud. He never lost the chance to tell the gullible that these were the stigmata of the Crucifixion. The examining doctor makes a note to show the Dupuytren's contracture to the medical students.

Day Twenty-one. A gray dawn slides through the ill-fitting slats of the venetian blind. From the glum faces of the nurses, it is clear that in the blockhouse things are looking worse. Whatever fragile equilibrium between acid and base, between oxygen and carbon dioxide, between positive and negative that the doctors have managed somehow to piece together has come unraveled. All of the vital signs have taken a turn for the worse. Fever. If it goes any higher, he will burst into flames. A pair of gills would work better than his solidified, liverish lungs. Daedalus! You can make anything! How about it? A pair of gills for the man!

"Let him not die," someone murmurs. The possibility itself lowers the temperature in the room; the patient shivers. With the sheet pulled down, he looks more and more like a winter-starved deer, stricken. *Don't go! Not yet!* Who is that calling out? Then I see that it is I calling out in pursuit of myself. The sheet is drawn smooth up to the armpits (as though he could move) and tucked under the mattress. When the nurse lets his head down, the pillow is scarcely dented by the weight of it. If someone had asked him at that moment what was his dearest wish, it would have been to lie on his stomach with his arms bracketing his head.

Day Twenty-two. All day and night, silt has settled in his veins, turning them solid. Only the bubbles of saliva on his teeth continue to wink bravely in the light. A slow slide of clot advances through his body. It began in the venules of the arms and legs, filled the larger veins, the iliac, the inferior vena cava, flowing slowly toward the heart. By morning, it will have achieved the right auricle. A single muffled thump, and it will be hurled to the lungs. And there it will stay, hardening into a cast of the pulmonary circulation. Should he die, will I too feel the cold mud in the marrow of my bones?

Day Twenty-three. And now it is my sad duty to report to you his death. It occurs at precisely 1:38 P.M. on April 23. He has been in the intensive care unit for three weeks and two days. From far away there comes a drumming so faint and rapid as to be unrecordable by even the most sensitive device in the room. Could it be rain? No, the sound lurches and staggers as though the drummer had slipped and lost his beat.

"Ventricular tachycardia," says the nurse and

calls for the doctor. The drumming grows louder and louder until it fills the room. Then all at once it stops as though an arrow had been shot through the throat of the drummer boy. The pace of activity in the room quickens. Maureen pounds vehemently upon his chest, turns up the oxygen flow. Injections are given into the tubing, then directly into his heart (or where she surmises his heart to be), syringes full of calcium and adrenaline. Electrodes are clapped to his chest and a series of jolts delivered which cause the body of the man to jounce hideously in the bed. His lips and fingernails are a deep blue. Minutes go by. The doctor arrives.

"How long has the EKG been flat?"

"Four and a half minutes." For a while they continue their efforts, which are like a pantomime. To no avail. No amount of resuscitation has the least effect. The heartbeat is not restored. At last the efforts are discontinued. There he lies, the sheet having been thrown off in the struggle, his slight body pale, emaciated, childlike were it not for that head like a Roman senator's and his aluminum hair.

"This man is dead."

Maureen, she who had pounced upon him like a cat, jolted him with currents of electricity, seen to the injections into his very heart, sags against a wall. She has given up trying to catch his ghost, which was running away from her. He was already out of her reach and she could not pursue him further. Sorrowfully, Maureen sits by the bed recording the events in the chart, her usually strong, bold hand-writing gone shaky. See how she pleats her forehead, draws in her lips, for in spite of all that she has wit-nessed over the years she cannot bear to be present at this. Time of death, she writes, 1:38 P.M.

It is strange, this painless death. Like stepping through a door held politely open for him. It doesn't seem right, somehow; a trivialization of the event. Death ought to be harder to achieve. Better to be hunted down, rooted out, hurting and bloody. Then death would come as a relief. It would be welcome.

. . .

IT IS NOW ten minutes since the doctor's pronounce-ment of death. Already the man has taken on that look of dignity that the newly dead have because of their possession of secrets. Or is it that they travel in a beyond that must be entered formally? Maureen is still writing an account of the last minutes of his life, her efforts to resuscitate him—the intracardiac injections of calcium and adrenaline, the jolts of elec-tricity delivered to his chest, the failure of the electro-cardiogram to respond. Glancing up, she has noted the characteristic "settling" of his body, the fixity that is incontrovertible; she has seen that so many times. Alone in the room, Maureen pauses in her charting to wipe her eyes with the back of her hand. Bleary with tears, she does not see what I see, that a subtle change is taking place in the contents of the bed, that the utter stillness of the body has been replaced by a calmness of the flesh, that beneath the closed eyelids his eyeballs roll slowly from side to side, then dart the way fish will move in a pond. Look! He shudders as if to shake off something which threatens to cling, and tightens those eyelids; minnows of light rising in the shallows. Then he hears a wingbeat, and feels something fugitive, immaterial, a beige veil being drawn from his face, slowly at first then faster, until the final whisk is like a slap. A moment later he draws the first breath. It is a deep sigh that might be interpreted as one either of sorrow or of satisfaction, as though one precious thing were being relinquished and another embraced. The nurse's incredulous stare! Her galvanic leap to his side! He, blinking in the explosion of light. When he opens his eyes, their color has gone from the ambivalence of hazel to the jubilation of blue.

Again, a breath is drawn, and another and another. A tracing has returned to the electrocardiograph, which the nurse had not yet detached from his arms and legs. The room, which had descended into a subaqueous silence emanating from the corpse, is now fiercely active. All the machinery is back in place, chugging, vibrating, clicking, ringing. Nurses scurry, calling out to one another. They bend over the bed, coaxing, noting and recording each sign of revivification. The intravenous chandelier sends light streaming through his body until he is something radiant and glowing in the bed. From time to time, the nurses turn to look at each other, their faces swept

with wild surmise. It is true! After ten minutes of cer-
tified death, this man has . . . risen. Risen! Such a
word does not belong in an intensive care unit.

Now the man is coughing against the endotracheal tube, he wrinkles his forehead, tears stream
from his eyes, he shakes his head slowly from side to
side. It is painful to observe the resurrection of a
man, to behold a log of inert flesh trying to raise itself. But the pain is all ours. He feels nothing as yet.
He is like the bulb of a tulip probing the earth in
which it has lain all winter unaware of its potential,
without memory or hope. As we do not ascribe pain
to the tulip in its rebirth so ought we not to imagine
that he, the man, is torn loose and abraded.

Then he who has performed no purposeful movement in three weeks reaches up one hand and pulls
the tube from his throat and mouth. And that is not
all: a smile breaks upon his face, but such a smile as
has never been seen on the continent of North
America. And in a hoarse whisper, but plainly
enough, he utters the single word: Yes.

"Did he say yes?"

"What do you suppose he means?"

"I couldn't say. Perhaps he was just answering a
question someone had asked him weeks ago before
he went into coma."

"Does that happen?"

"More likely it is some odd form of seizure
activity."

What he means, what the nurses cannot know, is that everything begins with a yes. That is how the first two bits of energy in the universe greeted each other, collided. Boom! And yes! There was life. So it is with the resurrected. Once again his throat fills with the word until the pressure of it is unbearable and he cries out in the hoarse voice that sticks to his jaws . . . Yes! Saying yes to life, accepting once again the burden and thrill of it.

• • •

IT IS THE NEXT DAY. He lies on his back, arms and legs splayed out so as not to disengage any of the needles or tubes. Now and then, he is propped on one side or the other. What he really wants is to curl up so as to give himself a hug, to accept his own warmth. Still, on his face is a strange, far-off look, as if to say, death is easy; it is the return to life that requires courage. When a nurse comes to take his temperature, he follows her solemnly with his eyes that seem to say: I have been to the land of the dead. Do not touch me. From that moment on, his vital signs—pulse, blood pressure, temperature—are normal. His oxygen saturation, 100 percent. There is no longer any doubt that he will recover.

About the consternation of the entire medical staff, there is little to be said. The joy at his reawakening is general, but in each person it is colored with uncertainty.

"You must have been mistaken," they tell the nurses at the weekly morbidity/mortality conference. "It cannot be as you told it . . ."

"The cardiogram was flat," the nurses reply. "The pulse and blood pressure were unobtainable. What else do you need? He was dead."

"Then how . . . ?" The nurses shrug and shake their heads.

Throughout the hospital they can think of nothing else. For weeks, in the laundry, at the coffee shop, in the X-ray file room as in the morgue, every conversation will begin with the words: Did you hear . . . ? On whatever flimsy pretext, orderlies and technicians and next-of-kin will walk past the doors of the intensive care unit just to draw near to the site, each of them taking away a dollop of hope to be saved up for a rainy day. If it happened to *him*, then perhaps . . . It is as if no one who worked at the hospital could go on living without specific knowledge of the event. Just so has it swollen into a legend that even I have come to believe in time. Such is the power of literature, be it written down on paper or passed on from mouth to ear.

· · ·

IT IS TWENTY-FOUR DAYS since the night he was taken to the emergency room, well into April. A warm day, with the sun streaming in and lighting up the wall of his room. Torpor envelops him. He hears grasshoppers. They seem to be in the bed with him, all around him, inside his chest. Yes! The noise of the grasshoppers is coming from inside his chest! He gives a soft, flannel cough and the stridulation abates. The ceiling at which he is gazing is made of squares of corkboard. Here and there the expanse of it is interrupted by the handle of an opaque glass panel that can be pulled down. Storage space. Or a hidden compartment like those in the ceiling of a ship's cabin. On board a ship you have to make use of every inch of space. He feels beneath him the gentle rocking of the sea. A coziness comes over him. He is perfectly comfortable. *So!* He thinks, *I am aboard a ship. But where? Perhaps I am in the South?* Yes, he remembers, it is the South; he had been there recently, lecturing in Texas. That's it, Texas! Then he sees the intravenous attached to his arm and he thinks that while in Texas he must have fallen sick, that he is aboard a hospital ship in the Gulf of Mexico. Doubtless soon to be discharged, from the way he feels. So comfortable and drowsy.

From somewhere comes the music of a Strauss waltz. He lies utterly still, letting the light from the intravenous chandelier trickle onto his face and collect there in small glistening pools, while the mattress takes up the rhythm of the music, scooping, dipping, turning his all but transparent body. He has never felt so graceful, so comfortable in his own flesh. All at once he has an irresistible urge to laugh. Should you ask him the reason for his laughter he would not know, for it is unlike any laughter of his life but something with which he has been infested, a holdover from some almost forgotten glee, now become reflexive and without rhyme or reason. He hears a woman's voice calling.

"Wake up! Wake up, sleepyhead! What's so funny?" It is as though she were summoning him up from a great deapth to the surface where he now floats between two sheets, his face visible only in the trough between the waves. He opens his eyes to see his wife, Janet, standing by the bed.

"For goodness' sake!" he says. "What are you doing in Texas, or off the coast of it?"

"This is not Texas," she informs him. "And this is no ship. You are in the intensive care unit of the Yale-New Haven Hospital."

"But the rocking of the waves . . ." He is not ready to give up.

"They have you on one of those newfangled mattresses that inflates here, deflates there. It's run by electricity. That way you won't get bedsores."

"How long have I been here?" It is the only thing he wants to know.

"About three weeks. Twenty-three days of coma to be exact." But he is already hurrying back to sleep.

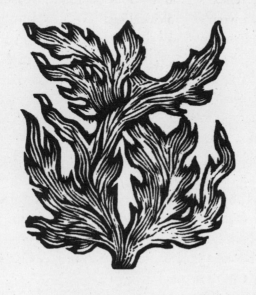

PART THREE

. . .

. . .

The stretcher bearing him to the infectious disease ward leaves the intensive care unit amid the applause and hoorays of the staff. Maureen stays with him until she is satisfied that he has been safely ensconced in his new room. When it is time for her to go, she roughly scrambles together the bright mane of her hair, then bends to kiss his cheek.

"You," he whispers, "all by yourself are enough to raise the dead." She lets out a whoop of laughter.

The ward to which he has been moved is occupied by other very sick medical patients, most with AIDS. The staff are largely Irish, brought to America because of the nursing shortage. They are men and women whose polite manners, wit, and soft brogue lend to the ward an atmosphere of old-world gentility. He, however, is to be psychotic for a time—the insanity, they say, is the aftermath of all the drugs and their withdrawal, the long coma, deprivation of sleep, and toxicity. It is confusing to go on thinking as a human after entering a world that is not. Like most forms of situational madness, it is aggravated by the coming of night. "Sundowning," it is called in the argot of clinical medicine. Later on, the hallucinations and delusions of this time are what will survive in his memory.

Once again the mattress upon which he has been deposited is divided into compartments that inflate and deflate in accordance with the electrical controls at the foot of the bed. While one compartment fills, another empties in a pattern which he is unable to solve. It seems to him capricious and mean-spirited. At one point in the cycle, it is the entire center that collapses while the head and foot rise as if to coapt, and he feels himself sliding into the abyss. In order to avoid that, he must cling all night long to the siderail of the bed, fighting off sleep until dawn, when the dreadful contraption will at last relent. It happens during the night that a nurse will try to pry his fingers from the siderail to which he is clinging for dear life. But he is like a parrot in a tree, at all times hooked to a branch by one of its feet or its beak.

Really, it would be cruel to make him let go, to

place him at the mercy of such a mattress. It is a predicament made all the more desperate by the fact that he cannot utter a sound; his vocal cords, held apart so long by the tube, do not yet approximate. He cannot call out. *Help!* is a word not available to him. What does emerge from his throat is little more than a hoarse gasp that is untranslatable to the nurses on the ward. Still, his lips never stop moving. With the sheet kicked away and his body exposed he could be a schoolboy huddling under a tree in a thunderstorm telling himself stories to keep his courage up.

Then too there is his eyesight, the lack of it. Amid the frenzy of that first night in the emergency room, his glasses had been lost, never to be found again. Now everything exists in a myopic haze. Once, opening his eyes, he saw a large, undulating mass at the foot of the bed. As he watched, it distended, quivered, elongated, then thinned out until there was only a narrow bridge of protoplasm joining the two halves. Then this too vanished and where there had been one, there were now two!—a doctor and a nurse—who walked away in opposite directions. Had he witnessed a mitosis? he wondered. An episode of binary fission? Add to blindness and muteness the atrophy of his body and you have a creature that is little more than a polyp on a stalk.

Only his imagination—driven by madness—roams far and wide. In the course of a single night he travels to a medieval monastery in 13th-century Ireland, where he undergoes a harsh novitiate against

his will. Minutes later he is in the delta of the river
Nile, wading among the fat, yellowish serpents that
are native to that region. From there, it is on to
Molokai on a tall sailing ship. Father Damien himself
comes out to greet him, the face of the holy man already bearing the leonine marks of his leprosy. It is
no wonder that by morning he is exhausted.

He awakens to the smell of lilac and rubbing alcohol. The lilacs sit in a urine specimen jar on the
sink; the rubbing alcohol is being spilled onto the
small of his back, then spread by a hand with the
consistency of pumice. A man speaks in an Irish
brogue.

"I'm Patrick, your nurse. I'll be lookin' after ye
from three o'clock to midnight every day."

"I've messed the bed. I'm sorry."

"We don't care about that here," Patrick replies.
"Besides, you don't have diarrhea, it's just incontinence. When you get stronger, it will take care of itself." So that is Patrick, with his talent for
forgiveness of the flesh. He is the sort of nurse who
can draw the pus out of a carbuncle with his gaze
alone, turn it into a jewel.

At this moment I, the authorial voice, should like
nothing better than to begin using the first person
pronoun, but madness, like coma, does not warrant
the pronoun *I*. And so I shall continue to act as inter-
mediary between the sick man and the outside world.
We have become something like identical twin brothers, only one step closer—joined about a single heart.

That accounts for my ability to convey what it was he felt in his coma and now his dreams, his hallucinations. It is only the independence of his illness that separates us. Illness causes one to go his own way unaccompanied. (Then again, the separation of our two bodies may be no more than a literary device. I can't say at this time.)

· · ·

WHEREVER DID the notion come from that flowers gladden the heart of the sick? The man has not been in his new room for more than an hour when there is delivered an ill-wrapped, ungainly parcel that, peeled down, proves to be an arrangement of seven tulips, all of the same waxen, corpselike shade of white. Immediately, the temperature of the room drops twenty degrees. They are the largest tulips of his life. A closer examination would have revealed that the long stems had been impaled on a bed of spikes and wired such that the distant hydrocephalic blossoms would respond to the least current of air. Placed on the window ledge, the evil heads are in a constant state of motion, nodding or shaking as if to vote yea or nay in the matter of his fate. At night the shadows of these flowers are magnified and thrown upon the wall—seven bald witches lunging for his thoughts.

It is the same each nightfall. He has been fed and bathed and made ready for sleep. His body, however, is not relaxed, but rigid, a corpse with its feet side by side, its eyes wide open. How does he feel? Midway between fear and despair. There is only one way to go after all: forward. Might as well put one foot before the other and march. Yet with pistol drawn and ear cocked. Oh, he would rest as he has been commanded to do, but he would not lie down. Oh no! Only squat with knees on chin. The better to stand and run.

There they are! On the wall! Sheeted by the moon, those caricatures of tulips, hunchbacked, swollen. Already, hunger stirs the mattress from its sleep. He can feel the rumbling of its bowels. Soon the dreadful peristalsis will begin. He reaches for the siderail, clutches it tightly. The night's long vigil has begun.

Ssshh! It is midnight at the Abbey of St. Ronan. Listen!

I am writing this in the scriptorium of the Abbey of St. Ronan in the hopes that one day this manuscript will be seen and the truth about my situation become known to the world. Doubtless it will be too late for my good, but there is the satisfaction of hope. It is a year ago that I was brought to this desolate monastery against my will. For surely, I have no calling to the religious life, only a handful of superstitions which do me just fine, thank you.

The truth is that I love sin. Folly, disgrace, scandal—the whole place caving in. Fiasco. If there is any sin available here, I haven't found it (that may be a lie). I was a gift to the abbot from the lord of the feu-

*dal states where my father is gamekeeper; this, in re-
turn for certain indulgences in the next world.*

*The Monastery of Şt. Ronan stands at the very
edge of a cliff overlooking the Irish Sea. From the
open boat, with a bitter wind tossing the ocean's
white hair, it is little more than a pile of battered
rocks. I am here because from childhood on, the old
priest who was the private confessor of my lord
taught me Greek, Latin, and the art of lettering—at
all of which I have become something of a master. I
spend most of my day and half the night in the scriptorium, the only place where my lack of piety is toler-
ated. (I make no secret of my opinion of the monastic
life.) It is often said by the older monks who sit side
by side with me that, had I remained in the world, I
should have made a passable surgeon, so sure and
steady is my hand with the stylus. It's true. Even with
a badly carved pen and raw parchment, I write and il-
luminate more beautifully than any of the others.*

*My only pleasure, aside from the pride I take in
my work, is the evening stroll in the cloister. At least
it used to be. Until recently, when another novice,
Gunther, has taken to badgering me during that
hour, the only time when conversation is permitted.
Gunther, damn him, is far too handsome—olive skin,
black eyes and hair, a row of even white teeth. And
the falsest smile in Christendom. Add to that a narrow, lewd, down-curved nose and a wide mouth. I
should have guessed him to be a Spaniard, but I
know he is the nephew of the abbot, a black*

Irishman if ever there was one. Since no one is allowed to remain alone lest he slip into solitary error (you know what I mean), we are paired off even for choir and recreation. Wouldn't you know? A hundred monks in his place and I get Gunther with his smiles and that voice all furred with malice. He is a fanatic, wants to be a soldier for Christ, and he never loses a chance to mock my underdeveloped bump of reverence.

Listen to this: at the north end of the cloister there is a kitchen garden. Bees are kept there as well. The other night as we strolled past, Gunther reached into a hive and drew forth a fistful of bees, which he stuffed inside his habit. When I cried that he would be stung, he sang out in good cheer that he longs for it with all his heart so that he might "offer it up." You should see his little bag of whips. (Damn this pen! Must I carve them all myself?)

In spite of all that zeal, no halo swings above his head (nor is it likely to). Only the dark flame of his black and passionate hair. But about that, I shall close my mouth upon the pill of silence. I do not carry tales. Instead, I tell Gunther that he is not to feel guilty; he is not to blame for the restless blood of the Crusaders in his veins. It is obvious that he is the favorite here. Even in a monastery, beauty has its own prerogative. Never mind, my parchments will mellow for a thousand years. Who will remember Gunther and his bees?

· · ·

Noon. It is hot as only Egypt is hot. Once again, I am standing in the mud of the delta. All about my legs slither—singly and in knots—venomous yellow asps, each one fat, heavy, and with a flattish penile head. I must not make even the smallest movement lest they attack. Steam rises from the Nile. Mangoes rot in the rich mud. There is nauseating smoke from fires made of camel dung. Dark red roses growing in silt. The delta of the river Nile.

Numerous barges and caiques sail downstream, the men standing idly in them. Having discharged their duties upriver, they are returning home. Free of the task of loading and unloading, they squat on the decks smoking and singing. Now and then, one will point to something on the banks—there! I follow his finger and see a group of women on their knees, dipping and pulling long strips of cloth in the water.

From four o'clock on he waits for the pigeons on the outside window ledge to awaken. Staring with myopic eyes, at last he makes out—just barely—the soft grayish mounds rising and settling as the sleeping birds are nudged by the dawn. Thank God! It is almost daylight. He could not have borne much more of this night.

Janet arrives with a large-faced clock. She places it on the window ledge next to the tulips.

"Part of the trouble," she says, "is that you don't know what time it is. And, if nothing else, the ticking will restore you to life in the morning."

"What are you talking about?"

"You're . . . ah . . . wandering? You know, sometimes you do . . ."

The words of the speaker come garbled to his ears. He must reach after them, sound them out phonetically in order to make sense of them.

His three children, all fully grown, are standing at the bedside, shell-shocked. He knows that look on their faces. It is the same look as when, twenty years ago, one of them had fallen down and needed to be picked up and consoled. It is one thing to see a father in coma; it is entirely another to behold his madness.

"Stop staring at me," he orders them. He tries clearing his throat but it remains a hank of gray tatters.

"Don't you know a person gets weak from being stared at?" It touches his heart to see six eyelids lower as one in an act of filial piety. Voiceless, he delivers a sermon with his eyes, producing the words all across his face where his children might read them.

The subject is filial piety. The text: Genesis 9:20, the drunkenness of Noah.

Noah drank too much wine and while he was drunk uncovered himself inside his tent. One of his three sons, Ham, saw his father's nakedness and told his two brothers outside to come and look. Instead Shem and Japheth took a cloak, laid it on their shoulders, and entered the tent walking backward. When they reached the place where Noah lay, they let fall the cloak so as to cover their father. Only then did they turn around to look at him. Every man, he preached, should have sons like Shem and Japheth.

"You're always saying sons," says Gretchen with her beautiful, sulky eyes. "As if I weren't a girl."

"Oh, my Gretch . . ." He tries to tell her but it won't come out. He has run out of voice.

Rounds. The room is crowded with people peering down at him. A perfect stranger pulls down the sheet that covers him. What is he looking for? His toes? Yes, he cups the patient's heel in his hand, presses and releases the toenails one by one. All the while, the doctor is lecturing to the students. Another stranger bends above an antecubital fossa, sniffing, he supposes, for a vein.

"There aren't any left," he tells her. "You are too late."

"You have to start eating," says another. "It is time to become anabolic again." He waits for the doctors to leave.

Patrick enters carrying a tray.

"Lunch," he announces (he pronounces it *loonch*). "A loovely word. Makes me salivate just to say it." He pours milk over a bowl of gruel, makes as if to assist the patient, who gags audibly. "So that's it, is it? Well, if ye won't feed, I must administer one way or t'other. Which'll it be today?"

"Here, I'll do that," says Janet. She rummages in her bag, brings forth a long wooden spoon.

"The never-fail family feeding spoon." She brandishes it. "More gall? More wormwood?" she asks gaily.

She advances the spoon toward his mouth, opening her own as if to show that love and gruel are somehow related. The man pretends to have fallen asleep. "Stop that!" he is scolded.

"Hag," he mutters.

"I am rather, aren't I?" she says brightly. "Open your mouth."

And in goes the wooden spoon.

"The food in this monastery stinks," he tells her.

"For the tenth time, you can't possibly be in a monastery, not with me here. They don't allow women." It is not sympathy in her voice, nor any hint of indulgence as though he might be a child that needed to be assuaged. No, it is more like endurance, acceptance. The man opens his eyes, recognizes her.

"Oh, it's you! What in heaven's name are you doing here?" He sleeps. When he awakens, he is alone. The sickroom is filled with the air of renunciation and obedience. His desire is to be released from it. How much easier to have yielded to the languor, gone limpsy-dewsy into death. No need then to swallow the repulsive food; no carnivore mattress; no yellowish asps. Gone too that militant novice with his mockery and his little bag of whips. It is not death that he hates; it is this borderland between, where terror and discomfort prevail. To return to life is to embark upon yearning again.

Midnight. I have just left Khartoum—a narrow escape—and am poling the caique upstream, the wooden rudder cleaving the mummy-brown water. All along the banks, in the moonlight, I see the white necks of motionless ibis questioning among the papyrus. From the shore drifts the nauseating odor of burning camel dung. Torture, bribery, flogging: that's the way things get done in Khartoum. A more miserable and unhealthy place can hardly be imagined. Dead animals rotting in the river, billions of flies and mosquitoes, the sewage of several nations floating in the current; fever, deceit, and crocodiles that can turn their heads around to look at you. And, of course, the yellowish asps with their flat penile heads. Now and then on of these will distend itself like a bladder and burst, scattering its venom, drops of which fall on the deck of the caique.

"Salaam aleikum!" I am hailed from another caique. "Baksheesh! Baksheesh!" comes the cry for alms. I dare not respond lest one of the beggars prove to be a murderous thief. So desperate are they that one or more will swim out to cling to the side of the boat, risking the asps and the crocodiles. It is well known that the Nile demands a human sacrifice for every passage upstream . . . Meanwhile, word has come that I have been reported dead and that the Royal Society is even now mounting an expedition to search for my remains, to solve the mystery of my long disappearance . . .

. . .

The doctor arrives. His name is Gordon.

"Well, where is the world traveler now?"

"Far up the Nile," says Janet. "Just passed Khartoum, I believe. A filthy place, with carcasses rotting on the riverbanks, a hundred billion flies, and crocodiles that can turn their heads and look at you."

"I didn't know crocodiles could do that."

"Only the ones in the Nile."

"How are *you* getting along?" the doctor asks her.

"This madness," she asks, "how long will it last?"

"I hope not much longer. It's the aftermath of the drugs and their withdrawal, the long period on the respirator, his own overheated imagination. And now the fever. Still, think of it this way: he has come a long way."

"If you think madness is an improvement over coma."

"This is no time to get discouraged."

"No."

"Get him to write down all his nightmares and hallucinations."

"Write them down! He can't even hold a pen."

"I mean get him to describe them to you so you can copy them down. Then you can read it all back to him later on. It's a way of splicing dream to reality. Sooner or later, he'll get the idea. I'll tell the nurses to do it too."

"I wish he would forget about that damned monastery. That's the one that bothers me the most. Actually, I rather like the Nile. Its gets downright exciting, what with all those close calls."

"Now that we've got your body under control, we'll have to work on your mind," says Patrick. Then to Janet: "What do ye suppose the hallucinations mean?"

"I know why the Abbey of St. Ronan and why Molokai."

"Tell me."

"The street we live on is named St. Ronan Terrace. Once, at Christmastime, he wrote an amusing account of the life of the ancient Celtic saint of that name. He sent the boys around to deliver a copy to each of the neighbors. Also, now and then, for all his blabbing about atheism, he goes to stay with the monks for a while; says he likes to be in the vicinity of piety. The fact is that there is a good deal of monk in him. In another century I suspect he could have ended up as one."

"And Molokai?"

"Two weeks before he got sick, he'd been on the island of Kauai giving some lectures. One of the people there had written a biography of Father Damien and had given him a copy. He was reading it the day before I sent him here in an ambulance."

"That leaves the river Nile."

"I have no idea where that one came from. He

surely does get around—from Hawaii to Egypt to Ireland, back and forth across the years. As though his bed is a magic carpet."

He travels through the void at immense velocity. Where he is, there is no friction, no inertia, no resistance. It is in madness as it is in coma—no passport required. The bed is more a hippogryph than a magic carpet, one of those mythic beasts—half horse, half winged griffin—that, once mounted, can fly anywhere in the world in minutes. It is the way the sick travel far and wide without moving from the bed.

In the room, someone is whispering. "What do you think, Pat?" It is his wife asking.

"I'd estimate his horsepower at twenty-five. Might do ten miles an hour on a flat stretch. But you know . . . it all begins to fit together somehow. Saint Ronan, the scriptorium, me an Irishman, the abbot and doctor interchangeable. Those dreams and hallucinations—they do have an odd logic to them. I wouldn't be surprised if he's hanging on tight to those dreams of his for some reason. Perhaps he's looking for clues to find the road back."

And now it is the doctor once again explaining to Janet: "There are a number of causes for it." He tells her about the effect of hypoxia on the brain, the alterations in biochemistry, the breakdown of cellular protein, the interruption of synapses. She nods and shrugs. But he is wrong. It is nothing of the kind. It is imagination; it is dream. Hallucinations. What are they if not the wreckage of submerged realities?

Damien is barefoot. He lifts and gathers his cassock in one hand before stepping into the waves to greet me. The gesture is graceful, almost feminine. Then I see that the fingers of the other hand, the one he raises in greeting, are absent, only blackened stumps.

Yesterday in a corner of the marketplace, I watched as a dozen Nubian girls, each about eight or nine years old, were sold for sixty pounds apiece. The ones who don't die of diarrhea along the way will end up in the harems of the sheiks in Arabia. Three young boys, too, who will be castrated and sent to the same destination. Just as the auction ended, my presence was detected and I barely escaped with my life. Several shots were fired. And now once again I am poling up the river.

"He isn't the only one." It is a young nurse, Robin, talking to Janet. "The whole ward is hallucinating. It's weird." As if someone in a laboratory is making mirages and releasing them here as vapor.

Afternoon. Warm day in late April. The patient is dozing on and off. A woman announces that it is time to eat. By the tone of her voice she intends to see to it. Within minutes he is being fed.

"I hate gruel."

"It isn't gruel. It's cream of mushroom soup." The voice of the woman is familiar.

"Get me a pen, please, and some paper. Get me a pen! Or am I not allowed to write? Where is the abbot? Let me up! I want to see the abbot!" It is the woman's turn to cry. He seems to her ever more haggard, emaciated, yet fighting like the devil in the bed. Who would have thought he had so much strength left in him, to struggle with, to punch? She backs out of reach of his flailing arms, weeps for his chattering teeth, his hands that tremble, less at this moment from fever than from a kind of rapturous haste to get somewhere, to reach a destination. She cannot know that what he wants to get away from is his own body, stretched out, drenched in sweat and urine, smelling of decay, unshaven, with liquid stool in the sheets. Once again he gathers his fury and calls out to her.

"Get me clean parchment, a stylus, ink. The abbot has instructed me to write down my dreams."

"Just a minute," says Janet. "I have brought it all—your notebook, a pen." She helps him to get a grip on the pen, but he cannot.

"Well, you can't hold it yet. Don't be upset. It's nothing to cry about. Look, now we are both crying." She laughs. "We'll try again tomorrow."

"Visitors to see you," says a nurse. He asks his wife to leave the room. To one after another of the newcomers he struggles to tell in his tattered-cloth voice how he is being held prisoner, that he is being force-fed, that he is being treated like a child. He begs them to intercede with the abbot. From their expressions, he knows that they have been instructed to indulge him. His wife is the only one he could trust. And now even she . . .

Still later, alone and forsaken, he will peer down the sheer face of the cliff at the base of which crashes the Irish Sea. He cannot possibly climb down without a rope or a ladder.

Dusk. A nurse has finished settling him for the night.

"Sweet dreams," she sings and flicks off the light.

"Tear their heads off!" he calls after her. But she has already left and cannot hear his frantic whisper. On the wall, the tulips bow and nod. Another night at the Abbey of St. Ronan.

Really, it is quite remarkable that it ever was built in such a place and with so much devotion. The stone, quarried from the cliff itself, rough-cut, squared, then set into interlocking patterns so as to make walls and arches. These arches, mutilated by centuries of wind and rain, are held up by square columns. The stone itself is a light warm ocher that goes gray at twilight. The sun seems to endow it with all the colors of the rainbow.

I have developed a fever. In the airless dome of the scriptorium a suffocating heat gathers. My sweat stains the parchment which then will not hold the ink. My hand shakes so that I cannot keep the stylus steady. In addition to that, I am being watched. All because of a few harmless pranks. Tiny venial sins. But around here that is grounds for being burned at the stake. The abbot, whom I had thought a fairly decent sort, turns out to be a fanatic of the worst stripe. Between him and Gunther, it is like the burning of the heretics.

By the way, I was wrong. The abbot is a Spaniard. His name is Tomas de Torquemada. A cruel name—has a ring of steel about it. However did he get himself assigned to an Irish monastery? Rumor has it that as a young monk Don Tomas was given the stigmata of the Crucifixion. Upon his ascension to the abbacy here (as the story goes), he asked Christ to conceal his wounds so as to discourage worship of his person. I'll bet! I don't know about any of that but this morning after visiting me in the infirmary, when he raised his hands in benediction, I could see bunched yellow scars on each of his palms, so maybe it is true. But I shouldn't be surprised if they were self-inflicted.

The sixth bell. Abruptly, Gunther sinks to his knees, approximating his palms beneath a bowed chin, and begins to pray. But I mean pray! His voice is strong, young, clear, his eyes dark as black olives; little drops of saliva gather at the corners of his mouth. Now and then he pauses, cocks his head as if listening, then resumes his murmur.

Look at that Gunther, will you? Easy to see that he's the favorite here. But I've got the goods on him and if it comes to that, I'll . . . If, as some say, celibacy makes one plump, he should be fat instead of lean. Well, well! Think of that! Think of that!

"Let me out of here! Let me out!"

"Now, now, stop that shouting. In a few days when your fever goes down and you no longer need the oxygen and when you start eating, you can go home. It doesn't help to shout and cry and use up your air."

"No, listen to me. Are you the one in charge here? I'm a scribe, not a monk. All this mortification of the flesh, the cincture, the fasting, it's not for me. Please let me out of here. I want to see the abbot. Take me to the abbot! I know my rights!"

At last, at last. Dawn, is it? The walls grow gray, then alabaster white. The tulips no longer cast their shadows but seem to be kneeling like monks on the window ledge, doing penance. And well they might! What is that familiar smell? For heaven's sake! Sandalwood! He remembers that they used to burn incense in the whorehouses in Troy. It smelled just like St. Peter's on Sunday. He remembers sitting there after Mass, when the priests swung the censer in the aisles, how he had had thoughts of a decidedly unholy nature. He tells that to Patrick who splits his sides laughing.

At precisely eight o'clock the abbot is standing by his bed.

"Well, how are we today?" he asks, using the papal plural. The man does not reply. "Anything we can do for you?"

"Father Abbot!" he clutches at the sleeve of a habit.

"We"—he might as well use the plural too—"are in lotus land. Help us!" The abbot takes a stethoscope and listens to the man's chest.

"Clear as a bell," he announces. The man must make the abbot understand. He must!

"Look, Gordon, Father Abbot, I think . . . I think I'm in lotus land."

"What's that? What did you say?"

"Don't go!"

"I'm not going anywhere. Tell me." He bends an ear until it is almost at the patient's lips, so as to hear.

"Lotus land," the patient says into the ear which has been presented to him. "First there's the monastery and the delta of the river Nile, then it's off to Molokai to visit Father Damien." The doctor straightens, gives the man a searching look.

"He's having nightmares," says the nurse.

"Oh! You're having bad dreams. Lotus land. The land of the lotus eaters. Now I get it!" Thank God! Thank God! What a sick person wants more than anything else is to be taken seriously.

· · ·

NOTE IN CHART: Lungs remain surprisingly clear although patient's respirations are still labored, shallow, and rapid. Fever and diarrhea persist. Worrisome. Patient states he is still in "lotus land," wherever that is. Benadryl prescribed at hour of sleep.

It takes an immense effort each time to hoist himself to the level of communication. By the time he has pulled himself up hand over hand to call for help, it is usually too late. He is terribly embarrassed by his incontinence. When it happens, he is sure he can see nostrils narrowing in judgment of the mess. He is wrong about that, of course. Dead wrong. No one cares; no one is shocked or disappointed. But tell that to a man like him who on his best days was painfully self-conscious, fastidious.

On all sides save the one facing the sea, the abbey is enclosed by a gray stone wall. It is of such a height that the top cannot be seen for the clouds that settle upon it. Often in my misery, I walk along this wall. Between the stones small ferns and tiny red geraniums are growing. I wonder what nourishes them? There is no soil, only the mortar that holds the stones in place. Perhaps it is something in the air that is absorbed through their leaves and fronds. Mosses too, of a bright emerald green, spread upon the stones, and lichen of various shades—orange, blue, grayish. From the other side of the wall, voices! Two women are speaking:

"Why doesn't he just find the gate and climb out?"

"Wouldn't you think so? It's so easy to do, but of course, he doesn't know."

The gate! So there is a gate! I don't remember having passed through it when I first came to St. Ronan. Had it been a dark night? Nor have I ever seen it since. I run along the wall searching for the gate. I run for a long distance before I must stop, panting and with my chest as though in a vise. Then I lean my cheek against the stone wall. A patch of moss—soft, cool, damp—offers itself to me. I move my head so that it is cushioned on the moss. I cannot find the gate. But I see it in my mind—a huge bronzy construction with two halves that would swing open to let a man out. The top is elaborately carved and ornamented, like a child's idea of the gates of heaven. Where is it? I must find it! I must! Now, from outside the wall, comes the wail of a woman. It is a banshee. I know it at once, waiting outside and wailing for the one who is about to die. Who could that be? The night my beloved old teacher lay dying, one of them was seen just outside the window of the room where he lay. Like all banshees, she was drawing a comb through her hair.

"Nurse! Nurse! You out there, please, I need the nurse! Help me! I'm dying!"

• • •

Awakening to the sound of bells, he wonders who has died. Best not to ask. It could be himself.

He is aboard a ship. There is the laughter of gulls, strident, harsh, the dipping of oars. What is it that he is supposed to do today? He can't remember. And then it comes to him—nothing. He is the one who is free of all human responsibilities.

Three times a day women (no, two of them are men) come in pairs and bathe him, a leg and an arm each. The torso is shared, one taking the chest, the other the back. They strip the sheets from the bed, replacing them with clean, sweet-smelling linen, pulling it tight so that there will be no wrinkles to bruise the skin. They turn him side to side in order to free the soiled bedclothes. Then he is dressed in a garment that snaps around the neck and arm, a johnny shirt. He lies between the two, yielding up to hands and cloths and lotion. He enjoys it as an infant must enjoy having its diaper changed. Each time, there is the sense of starting afresh.

Now and then it happens that even before they have finished, he soils the clean linen and they must do it all again. This they do without the least murmur, although he is in an agony of shame and self-disgust. Long after they have left the room he feels the warmth of their thighs, biceps, their breasts.

NOTE IN CHART: Patient continues to hallucinate about an Irish monastery, the Nile River, and

Father Damien. Seems to have some insight into his mental situation.

Khartoum, Molokai, St. Ronan—to each of them he travels by candlelight. Everything is enhaloed by a bright ring beyond which there is the seething darkness. Precisely because it is dim and flickering, he sees more than were there wattage in the thousands.

Look there! On the Nile, a boat of cypress wood drifting; the river itself brimming; boatmen calling out and beckoning to those who would cross to the other bank; deep black pools where floats the silver lotus; light glancing off the papyrus.

Strangely, he would not trade places with anyone else even if it were offered to him. No matter how dire his condition, he wants to be himself. It is the profound egotism of the human being. Nor does he wish to waste time asking himself: who am I? Or, what am I? He knows very well both to his shame and his pride who and what he is. Nor does he even once think about God. Whatever else has changed, his atheism has remained unshaken, thank God.

Each morning a woman comes to draw his blood. She is the shape and color of an eggplant. His veins, the lack of them, are her Calvary. She has needled his arms many times to no avail.

"Must we go on in this vein?" he asks her.

Unsmiling, she applies the tourniquet, shakes her head sadly. It is clear that she hates to do it.

"Your veins, they all used up. They ain't any more."

"No, they ain't," he agrees. The woman moans and he sees that her sorrow is genuine.

"Oh, go ahead," he tells her and turns to gaze out the window, willing himself to a distant land. The woman takes a large insect from a leather bag and lays it on his arm. There is a sharp sting. But by now, like Gunther, his flesh has grown contemptuous of pain.

"They all used up," the woman sings to herself. She runs her finger with obvious greed over his extensor pollicis tendon.

"No, no," he says. "That is a tendon, not a vein. Of all the tissues of my body, it is the least likely to contain what you are after."

"I knows, I knows."

"I am unclean," he says. "Whosoever toucheth my carcass shall also be unclean. Whosoever beareth away aught from my carcass must wash her clothes and bathe right away."

"Sweet Jesus!" calls the woman softly. "Keep me safe!" After half an hour of probing, she trips over a small vein. The blood runs down his arm.

"Hurry!" he tells her. "It will attract the rats."

"Oh, Lord Jesus!" she whispers. "Don't talk like that."

• • •

Just outside the door, the laughter of women. Two nurses enter the room, stand on either side of the bed. They remove his johnny shirt, strip the soiled sheets from his bed, turning him this way and that. All the while that they bathe him their laughter passes back and forth over his head. He cannot make out what they are saying. Now and then, one of them glances down, then rollicks off into another spasm of hilarity. One of them, Robin, is young, and vivacious. Is that a dark red scorn painted on her mouth? He decides yes, it is.

"Something funny about me?" he asks her. Once, in Fort Worth, Texas, he had been taken to a museum to see a collection of Cycladic art. It consisted of tiny white marble figurines, tomb ornaments used by the ancient inhabitants of the Aegean Islands. Each one a dead white color and with shoulders hunched, arms and legs thin and stumpy, eyes staring straight ahead. It seems to him, looking down at himself, that he has become one of them. A piece of statuary picked up on one of the Cyclades islands.

"You are laughing at me!" The young nurse stops her toweling, leans directly over his face. She is deadly serious now.

"Listen to me. There are not too many people here laughing at you or at anyone else. If we laugh, it is *for* you, not *at* you, so that you might hear it and be reassured. Perhaps it will be contagious and you will laugh too. If we are laughing, it is because we have to. If you worked here, I bet you'd laugh too."

Later, the nurse, Robin, and he discover that they are both from Troy, both born and raised there.

"I might have known," he tells her. "Troy, where every woman is a seeress, every man a warrior."

"Make that a whore and a drunk," she replies, "and I'm with you."

"Well, that too," he admits. They laugh together.

NOTE IN CHART: Patient expressing paranoid ideas. Thinks the staff is laughing at his body. Strongly disabused of this notion.

At 7 A.M. the maid arrives. Her name is Violet. She has the habit of humming to herself—tuneless, monotonous, held in, haunting.

"What's that you're humming?" he asks her.

"Hummin'? Was I hummin'? Oh nothin'. Just makin' a sound."

But each morning he reaches out to lock himself to the strange, rich noise she makes unconsciously and that has all by itself a healing quality. It confirms his suspicion that true healing is done through song and persuasion. As for his own voice, when the occasional remnant of it returns to him, he speaks in fragments, embryos of sentences, abandoning them almost at once, as though whatever it is he wants to say isn't worth the effort. Still it makes him weep out of frustration.

"What are you crying about now?"

"Tears," he croaks, "idle tears. I know not what they mean."

Two women are talking in the corridor. He, sly fox, has turned his face to the wall. He might be asleep, but he is not.

"How is he today?" That one's Janet, he thinks.

"Are you sure he isn't Irish?" The other is Robin, the Woman of Troy.

"Quite sure."

"The more you try to hide it, you know, the more it shows."

"What now?"

"Oh, he's full of the usual Trojan malarkey."

"Now what? Tell me."

"Something about Elizabeth I, that she was a boy?"

"Oh, not that old thing again. He didn't tell you that one. Say he didn't!"

"I didn't get much of it. He ran out of voice. How does it end?"

"The story goes that Elizabeth was murdered as a young girl and a lookalike boy substituted. That, he tells everyone who will listen, is why she a. looked like that; b. never married; and c. swore like a trooper."

"And he told that when he was sane? Who would listen?"

"Only the children when they were young. Here they come now. Your father's getting better—practically back to normal. Told the one about Queen Elizabeth." The way they all laugh . . .

"Eat! You must eat!" Each day and many times each day he is bidden to eat.

"Say farewell to catabolism. You must eat in order to live." But to eat without the blessing of hunger cannot be done. A dietitian comes to discuss his preferences. She is very pretty and plump. Together they will make out a menu for the next day, the correct proportions of fat, carbohydrate, and protein. He expresses his surprise that with all the advances in science there are still only those three categories. Her laughter goes all the way up the chromatic scale, like the song of a prairie warbler.

"I can live for a week on a tenpenny nail," he tells her.

"We aren't getting anywhere," she reminds him. "What would you like for dinner tonight?"

"For dinner? A glass of champagne in a crystal goblet and a single green pea." Then she takes charge.

"Fish," she says. "Chicken." The man gags at the sound of the words.

NOTE IN CHART: Patient refuses all food, states that his brain feels like a cheese—"Roquefort, ripe and falling to pieces."

· · ·

Midmorning: he must have dozed off. He opens his eyes to see Gordon standing at the bedside.

"Good morning," the doctor sings with the peculiar enthusiasm of the medical profession for happy greetings.

"It is and it isn't."

"I think you are well enough to be told the facts. I'm going to try to answer your questions."

"Questions?" He tries to think what is expected of him and cannot. How can it be that a lifetime of treating the sick has not prepared him at all for the role of the patient?

"Don't you want to know what was wrong with you? Your diagnosis?"

"Oh, yes! Of course I do. What was wrong with me? What *is* wrong with me?"

"We don't really know." The voice turns lame. The man remembers that in the medical profession one always dilutes responsibility for ignorance with the plural pronoun *we*.

"No diagnosis?" So, then. Death, had it come, would have worn a mask; it would have come anonymously.

"It's true. After all those blood smears, counts, X-rays, cultures—all the tests known to modern medicine—after all that, we are left with a diagnosis by exclusion. It couldn't have been anything else, so it had to be . . . Legionnaires' disease." He says the words importantly, as they deserve to be said.

"Legionnaires' disease? I'll take it. How did I get it?"

"All those air-conditioned hotels and planes. One of them may have been contaminated with *Legionella*. Can't tell."

"Pestiducts."

"Nice word. I'll have to remember that."

"What ward is this?"

"Infectious disease. Mostly AIDS."

"When I was ten years old, I used to read about the Foreign Legion in the Sunday rotogravure. There were pictures of the legionnaires riding camels across the desert, close-order drilling inside the dazzling white compound at Timbuktu. I died to be one of them."

"Well, it's fifty years later, and I guess you almost did."

"That bad, was it? Must have been, from the looks of what's left of me."

"There was just nothing we did not do to get you to wake up."

"Did you try tickling?"

"As a matter of fact your boys did try tickling you. You shivered, either with agony or delight, it wasn't clear. The reactions of the body are sometimes ambiguous."

For all of that, some of the monks are rather sweetly insane. My favorite is the gardener. Yesterday

at chapter he announced that under certain condi-
tions tea made of heliotrope petals can make you
invisible. He wouldn't say what conditions, and no,
there is no heliotrope growing within a hundred
leagues of here as it is a Southern flower. Once I
caught him exorcising the devil from a head of cab-
bage! Made me split my sides. The good man avoids
me ever since I told him that "paradise" comes from
the Persian word for garden.

Day after day he implores his doctor to discharge
him from the hospital. He yearns for home like an
exile, for his study, small as a nutshell and as brown;
for the house which sits at the top of a quiet steep
hill in the very center of the city. From the window of
his study he can look down upon an archipelago of
roofs, each one topped with one or two chimneys
and a weather vane, and each engulfed in the foliage
of large trees. Would he ever return?

"Send me home, please! I beg you on the knees
of my heart, as they used to say in the old days."

"You're still having trouble breathing."

"It's this room. It's too small for my lungs. 'As
pants the hart for the cold mountain stream, I gasp
for wide open spaces.'"

"Oh, that is good," says the doctor. "Very good.
How does it go again? As pants the heart . . . pants
the heart?"

"Hart—*h-a-r-t*—you know, the deer."

"As pants the hart for the cold mountain stream.

Very beautiful." He writes it in his notebook. "No.
The answer is no. I will not send you home."

"But why?"

"Because you are short of breath, because you
have fever, and let me be honest: you are still con-
fused, hallucinating."

"Isn't there an old remedy for it? Apply pigeons
to the soles of the feet. It draws the vapors down
from the brain. There are a dozen of them on the
window ledge at any given time."

"I don't want to have to worry about you, wonder whether you are okay. I need to have you here
where I can feast my eyes on what's left of you.
Maybe I've grown too fond of you?"

"You can visit me at home three times a day. You
can sleep at the foot of my bed. I'll pull your ears,
scratch your tummy. Let me go home!"

Of all the terrors that assail him during the endless nights, the carnivore mattress is prime. It is
shortly before midnight. For four hours he has fend-
ed off the mattress, his right hand fused to the
siderail the way a drowning man clings to a bit of
flotsam, and with the malevolent tulips nodding yes,
shaking their heads no. It is his tenth night on the
ward. He must get out of here! Transferring his grip
from rung to rung, he slithers to the foot of the bed.
Pulling himself to a sitting position, he drops his feet
over the side. Now he is wedged between the siderail
and footboard, unable to move either back onto the

bed or farther down from it. He calls out for help, but whatever voice he produces sticks to his jaws. Just as well. They would come, secure him hand and foot, deliver him up to the creature.

At last the mattress emits a deflationary sigh such that there is a bit of room. The man slips through to the floor. On the wall, the black shadows of the tulips wave in disapproval. It is the first time that he is free of the bed, standing! But the struggle has cost him dearly. He has gambled far beyond his means. He lurches to the sink and sees reflected in the mirror above it not a man, but a specter, an image of madness—mouth agape and huffing, the whites of his eyes visible all around the pupils. The nightshirt has become unstrapped from the struggle and hangs from one shoulder. "Help me!" he cries, but no sound comes.

He slides to the floor. Lying prone as in the muck of the Nile delta, he is unable to satisfy his hunger for air. Slowly, he advances one hand a fraction of an inch, then the other, into the empty darkness. His hands are the pseudopodia of an amoeba. Helplessly, he discharges from his excretory pore, feeling all of his granules blow this way and that. Suddenly the darkness produces a foot, then another. A man's feet in white sneakers. They are planted on either side of his head. In the long, shocked silence, he wonders whether the man is going to urinate on him. He himself at the moment is leaking away to nothing.

Click! And abruptly the room fills with light.

From on high comes a stern, reverberant voice.

"That was a stupid and dangerous thing to do. Just look at ye, sprawled." The amoeba shudders; its granules swirl about in a kind of protozoan weeping. There is a hand at his face. "Here's your oxygen. Try to breathe more slowly. Ye don't have to pant so. I'm here, and I'll look after ye now. No, no, I shan't leave, not to worry. Look up here; watch my chest and breathe along with me." The man lying on the floor looks up toward the source of the voice. It is a man wearing a blue scrub suit. He is thickset, and has a black beard going gray. He bends over the patient. "Here, give me your hand." He places the patient's hand on his own chest, holds it there, breathes emphatically. "In. Out. In. Out. Much better." He straightens now, his feet only inches from the sick man's head. The closer foot is tapping. When he speaks again, it is in a soft, flannel brogue that is utterly devoid of reproach.

"I'm your solution," he says.

"What?"

"I'm goin' to solve ye. Trow ye into the toob, that's what."

"The toob?"

"Aye, the toob." As if to clarify, he kneels and scoops the spent, mad creature from where he lies facedown in the muck of the Nile delta, lifts him as gently and precisely as a cat taking a kitten in its mouth. "Nothin' to ye—half a pail of coal, I'd say." He hefts the patient up and down in his arms. Now

they are in a small room entirely occupied by a bath-
tub and a wooden stool. "Fill 'er oop," says the
nurse and turns on the faucet, then peels off the filthy
raiment. Now and then he troubles the water with
his hand, which is large, burly, and undeformed by
the least elegance. The fingers are short and thick.
There is a dent in the thumbnail. He lowers his patient into the warm bath, which is to the sick man
like the pool of Bethesda from which the cripple
emerged whole. "It's like dippin' a sheep. To get rid
of the bugs and parasites.

"You're panting again. Slow it down. Breathe
when I do. Yes." With soap and washcloth, he bathes
the man, then scoops water with a plastic bottle and
pours it over his head, again and again. Now he rubs
lather into the man's scalp, massaging, rinsing. All
this while, the patient lies there, neutral, incurious,
breathing quietly for once. Nor does he feel the
writhing of his intestines.

"Ah, just wait till I get t'rough wit' ye . . ." From
where he lies in the tub he can see reflected in the
Irishman's face, ruddy and shining from the humidity, the satisfaction the man draws from his work. He
lifts his head, tries to look down at himself.

"What's wrong?" Patrick asks him.

"Hold me up. I want to see." He looks down at
his body, lets out a groan, falls back into the sup-
porting arm of his nurse.

"What is it?"

"My penis!" he says. The nurse casts a quick glance.

"What about it?"

"It's shrunk! Only a small button left. I knew I owed a cock to Asclepios but I didn't think it had to be my own."

"What are ye talkin' about?"

"Socrates, his last words—'I owe a cock to Asclepios.' He wanted to make sure the god was paid before he drank the hemlock." The nurse laughs.

"What's so funny?"

"Here all the time I thought ye were somethin' grand and come to find out ye're just another bloke worryin' about the size of his pecker."

At the end of a rare, sullen afternoon we have entered a natural harbor off Molokai. From the dinghy I see a small cluster of people on the beach. One, standing in front and a bit apart, wears a long black cassock and a broad-brimmed hat. Damien, I think. It is he. When he steps forward into the waves to greet me, I see the thickened tissues of his forehead and cheeks. I smell the putrefaction floating from his body; it is almost visible.

"I have been waiting for you," says the priest. "At last you've come."

Patrick leans over the man, leaning down as if to tell a secret.

"That is not true. Is it?" His voice, so gentle. And all at once, the man knows that it is not true. Only that it had seemed so.

"No," he says. "It is what I have made up." And a fresh wave of relief sweeps through him. He hadn't been to Molokai! It was just a dream.

"And all that about the river Nile? The swampy smell of the delta coating your tongue? Not true, right?"

"I have never been to Egypt."

"You have been telling stories. All right, then. We'll forget about it. No looking back. I'll miss our visits to the Abbey of St. Ronan, though. Just when they were beginning to get good. Gunther and his little bag of whips. Really now! Behave yourself!"

At last the sick man is lifted forth from the tub, clean, calm, and sane. Rubbed dry, he is carried back to his room. The hands of the nurse have the physical kindness of big hands, the way they form themselves into a nest. Settled into it, he could laugh out loud. Perhaps he will. He thinks of how, sixty years before, his father had carried him about in his arms.

"Now how do you feel?"

"Euphoric," he tells the nurse.

"You what?"

"*Phoric.* That means being carried. The *eu* stands for contented. I am happy to be carried." And he feels the heat and the strength of the solid man infusing him, entering his veins; his breathing lightens, his brain clears into a kind of bright amazement. It seems to him that his molecules, which had been in chaotic disarray, have rearranged themselves, fallen into place. It is the true moment of cure.

As for the rest? Well, that's just medical data. The part that can be read from a computer. That doesn't make you well. Arrayed in clean linen, he lies upon the bed.

"I turned the monster off," says Patrick, tapping the mattress. "Go to sleep."

Alone and content in his solitude, he raises one arm straight up in the air. Turning his head, he sees the gesture repeated in the mirror over the sink, only more slowly, with luxuriance and absolute comfort, as if his arm were floating in a warm, viscous fluid. The struggle, whatever it had been, is far away, too far to harm him. Had it been real? he wonders, then falls asleep.

Later, before going off duty, the nurse will write in the chart: 6 P.M.: patient remains anorectic, fed oatmeal by wife despite objections. Still unable to speak audibly. Embarrassed by diarrhea. Reassured on the score once again. At midnight, patient discovered lying on the floor of his room, severely dyspneic and incontinent of stool. He was in obvious terror, stated that the electric mattress "wants to devour me," that he has barely escaped with his life. Patient reprimanded for having gotten out of bed without permission. Given tub bath with good results. Breathing more quietly; pulse regular. Long story of how he sailed from the island of Kauai to Molokai in a tall sailing vessel to visit the leper colony, how he was met at the beach by Father Damien himself. Told to stop making up stories. He agreed. Sleeping peacefully.

I have been on the ward for two weeks. Every four hours a nurse appears with a handful of pills and capsules, glasses of medication. Each one as welcome as her taming was to Kate the shrew. Prednisone, erythromycin, Lasix, Benadryl, and what's that coffin-shaped tablet? Carafate, to coat your stomach. Metamucil, Pepto-Bismol, Lomotil, Bactrim. You could never mistake their names for anything else than drugs. Such a manufactured word—Pepto-Bismol—could never have been a flower. These nurses seem to speak in code. I cannot make out the meaning of what is said to me. The instructions are as if passed from mouth to mouth during a battle—*passe-paroles* that lose a portion of their meaning with each transmission.

So slowly and imperceptibly does the madness recede that when I go sane for keeps, neither I nor anyone else notices. By sometimes looking, by sometimes even not looking, I conjure the house on St. Ronan Terrace—the white paint peeling in great strips, the broken handrail, the deeply rutted driveway, the topless pine tree to the left of the front step, the lawn infested with yellow jackets, the moon coming down the staircase at night. It seems to me a far-off, be-

witched place where once I lived in peaceful symbio-
sis with my neighbors. Now, having been evicted, I
cannot find the way back. Ah! Just to think of the
crystal bowl on the dining room table in which
someone has floated Queen Anne's lace and the deep
blue flowers of myrtle; the paintings of birds on the
walls of my room—the pileated woodpecker, the
turkey vulture, and the puffin. The house and everything in and around it has a glassy air of being set
back out of earshot, in a time long past. I die to go
there, like a boy shut up in a hated boarding school;
to see home again would make me well.

Janet speaks to the doctor: "He wants to go
home, says he can't get well here, says if you don't let
him go, he'll sign himself out against advice." The
doctor turns to me.

"What do you need that you don't have here?
That we haven't given you?"

"Privacy. If I can't have that, I don't want anything."

"You do have a private room. What are you talking about?"

"I'm talking about solitude. A condition that does
not include people like you coming in here whenever
they feel like it and asking me what else I want."

"Aren't we touchy today?" Enter Patrick. "A regular leprechaun," he says.

"What's that got to do with it?" I have grown
huffy.

"The leprechauns were all shoemakers. Shoemakers are grouchy and cross. There's no expecting civility out of them."

"And you!" I am speaking to Patrick. "The way you have of coming into a sickroom like Justice itself, then moving around in it like Mercy . . . it isn't human."

"What else," says Patrick.

"That's it."

"What you have just heard," says Janet, "is my husband expressing *undying* gratitude."

"Go home then," says Gordon. "And good riddance. I'll arrange for the ambulance. Day after tomorrow."

"Tell them no sirens. I don't want to annoy the neighbors." The doctor turns away to indicate that he is no longer addressing me.

"I think it'll be all right. Get him to bed, feed him, see that he takes his pills. There'll be the visiting nurse to check him up and put him through some exercises. If you have any questions, call me anytime." Then there is Patrick taking up my hand from the sheet, holding it, pressed between both of his.

"You come back to see us, promise?"

It is the last day of my hospitalization. In the rooms on either side of mine, young men with AIDS lie in the extravaganza of death. They have eaten very little of the provender of life, poor boys. I imagine them tossing and turning in the restless industry of exhaustion. I listen to their febrile night cries that make no sense. How well I know that in the single combat with death, the mind is at best a slender adolescent squire, standing on the sidelines.

I awaken to the sound of strange music coming from somewhere down the hall, crystalline notes made on a hollow instrument such as has never been seen before. I imagine it made of black or dark green glass and equipped with a set of clappers. It must be played with the palm or the heel of the hand. The notes are sharp and clear. *Ping. Ping. Ping.* A lovely, cheerful melody. After each note women make appreciative small screams in Spanish. I see the dark shadows around their eyes, their languor, their large pelvises and breasts. I decide against mentioning this to anyone lest my discharge be canceled.

There are visitors. A young man with a pink slap permanently imprinted on his cheek enters the room carrying a flute. He is accompanied by a woman who sets pages of music on a stand. The young man lifts the flute to his lips. It is the Meditation from *Thaïs*, a piece of music that I have always hated. The young man is earnest. There is no escape. At last, it is over.

"Do you have any requests?"

"No." For God's sake, please go away! I don't actually say this but think it very clearly so that the flutist will see the sentence written on my face. For a long moment he looks at me sadly while the slap on his cheek deepens to crimson.

Next it is a rabbi wearing a long gabardine coat, a black fedora, and sidecurls. He is pale and pudgy.

He hands me a sheet of literature about the Hasidic sect of Jews. I tell him I would be as at home among the cannibals. Before I can stop him, the rabbi has placed his sweaty palm on my head and blessed me.

"*Yevorechachoh,*" and all that. No harm done, you say? On the contrary. Such an unwanted benediction is a form of molestation.

"Nice to meet you," the rabbi says and leaves.

In the afternoon, another musician! A woman with a violin.

"Anything you'd especially like to hear?"

"Do you know the Meditation from *Thaïs?*" When she has finished playing and left the room there is a long silence, after which Janet speaks.

"That was mean of you."

"Between the flute and the violin, give me the harmonica any day."

"Sometimes I think you are crotchety precisely because you have survived. Why else are you abusive to these well-intentioned souls?" I am silent. "No illness gives you the right to insult good people."

"I don't have to love everyone on sight, do I?"

"No, but you do have to be polite." All at once it is my own behavior that hurts. I reach out toward the door as if to call my victims back, to make amends.

"Quick! Run after them. Tell them I'm sorry. Ask them to come back for a moment. I want to say I'm sorry." I am full of shame.

"Oh, never mind, never mind. It is nothing to cry about. I'm sure they're used to it. A good thing you're going home tomorrow. You're as mean as a snake."

It is the morning of discharge. Three medical students are loitering in the corridor. First one walks by, peers in, then another. The last pokes his head through the doorway. I motion for them to come in. They have each brought a yellowed, dogeared copy of *Mortal Lessons*. Would I sign them? Yes, by all means. But the pen is turbulent in my fingers and won't hold still. The students watch my struggle in silence. I make three large X's.

"You know, before I went into the intensive care unit, I was right-handed. Now look! They've put me back together as a lefty." When they turn to leave, I collapse with relief upon the pillow. It is an hour before my discharge from the hospital. Gordon is paying a last in-house visit.

"The whole place is agog over your recovery."

"It's *your* fame that's spreading," I tell him.

"How so?"

"I'm telling everyone you brought me back from the dead. 'Get him in a good mood,' I say, 'and he'll do the same for you too.' But between you and me . . ."

"Yes?"

"Next time hold a feather to my lips. It's more reliable."

Dressed in my too-large clothes, I am waiting for the ambulance. Robin, the Woman of Troy, comes in.

"What do you like best about nursing," I ask her.

"Waving goodbye to the patients from the window."

"But goodbye . . . it's sad."

"In a hospital, it's the other way around. Hello is sad. Hello *again* is even worse. Goodbye is just right."

May 5: I am lying in my own bed at home. I look around to make sure. Yes, it is true! There are my bird drawings on the wall—the turkey vultures and the pileated woodpeckers.

"How did I get here?"

"You fell asleep in the ambulance. The men carried you upstairs."

"It is my fate to remember nothing, only to be told what happened afterward."

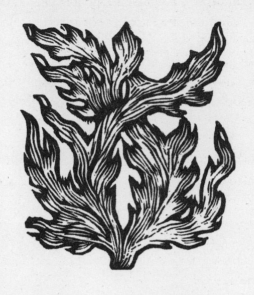

PART FOUR

. . .

. . .

May 10: I sit in the garden wearing a broad-brimmed straw hat. It is unseasonably warm, they say, but even with a woolen shawl over my shoulders I'm cold. A notebook rests on my lap; I am holding a pen. With a pince-nez on a long black ribbon, I could be Chekhov at Yalta. Every few seconds I cough. A small lung abscess has developed on the left, it seems, and a new area of infiltration in the right lung. Gordon visits.

"Maybe we need to do a bronchoscopy, a lung biopsy," he says.

"Maybe I'll just cough it up instead."

Now and then I write a few words in the note-book only to cross them out a moment later. Nearby, Janet, on hands and knees, is gardening furiously. Whenever the cough turns spasmodic, the trowel in her hand assumes the same rapid tempo. I am her consultant. Do I think the yellow iris clashes with the red azalea?

"That is *their* problem," I tell her. "I never take sides in disputes among the vegetable kingdom." The pen and the notebook are present out of habit and hope: habit because they have never been out of reach for twenty years; hope because I labor under the delusion that the mere setting down of words on a page—even such words as *and* and *the*—will counteract the atrophy of disuse. The sentences I write are of no value. They are simply exercises, like the ones I must do to rebuild my quadriceps muscles. Now and again I wonder about those three weeks in the intensive care unit of which I haven't the least recollection. Coma is a black pool in which one sees only his reflection.

This afternoon a woman came to visit. We sat in the garden. For an hour she looked at me the way one looks at a river flowing by. Then, when she stood up to go, she remembered to show me the enamel of her perfect teeth in a smile.

"So good to see you coming along," she said. "Now don't you ever dare to do that to us again."

June 30: It is the end of June, and still I sit in the garden pretending to write. What had been curiosity about those three weeks of coma has become an ob-session. *I want to know what happened.* I close my eyes and imagine my body given over to others for them to examine in all its particularities; perfect strangers who would come to know the ins and outs of my flesh the way they know the ins and outs of their shoelaces. Day after day I sit here waiting for the return of memory, but it does not come. Strange how, months later, those mad dreams will spring in-stantly to mind in all their lurid detail while the re-ality of coma remains hidden from me. Strain as I will, the membrane stays impermeable. It is no good asking others.

"You should be grateful not to know. Think of the kindness of nature in dropping a veil over all of that."

"All of what?"

"Whatever it is you say you need to know, for heaven's sakes."

"Tell me."

"Well . . . let's see . . . you were about as sick as anyone can be. You wouldn't have recognized your-self. Now just forget all about it. You're positively morbid."

But they are mistaken who would squelch the longing to know. Man's greatest pleasure is remem-bering. It's what makes us godlike, distinguishes us from the animals. Remembering is a way of reclaim-ing what was mine, what had been taken away from me. Forget it? Not likely. Janet changes the subject.

"So many yellow jackets this year! It's the lawn, gone half to clover. The bees love it." She makes a full circle around my chair holding aloft a can of insect repellent.

"If I were going to have a garden," I tell her, "it wouldn't be full of those vulgar day lilies."

"Oh? What would you have?"

"I'd plant flowers whose names mean something: sympathy, condolence, fit-of-pique."

"I'm not a bit surprised."

Come to think of it, the comatose brain is like a tree in winter, all its leaves gone, only a last year's nest remaining, high up. In May, a small scarlet bird will fly in and begin to sing rapturously. It will be spring; there will be leaves. Sooner or later he'll fly away. The tree will not remember the long sobriety of winter nor the drunken tanager.

Perhaps—I don't know—the helplessness of the sickbed, the amnesia, are more painful to a surgeon than to an internist, say, or a pediatrician. A surgeon is accustomed to authority; he is in control, he gives orders. After all, are we not the warriors of medicine who, taking up spear and shield, do single combat with disease? Hack away at it root and branch? Those others, they are the statesmen who deal diplomatically with the enemy: a little more digitalis, a little less insulin. How much harder for a surgeon is the return to an infancy when he must be changed, wiped, even restrained.

. . .

July 1: In the bathroom, stepping from the shower, I turn away from the mirror, from the sight of my sad shoulder blades, my ribs. One glance is enough to make me believe that I am somebody else, yet somehow recognizable. For the first time I see *why* transvestites go to such lengths to hide what they see as their wounds. I differ from them only in that I do not want to be looked at.

Patrick visits.

"They say that you are a saint," I tell him. "Is it true?"

"Certainly."

"Good! Then I'll know at least one person in heaven when I get there."

"Afraid not. Hell has to have its saints too, as well as heaven. I'm one of those."

July 5: I have decided to read my hospital chart. All through the holiday weekend I have waited patiently to phone the record room.

"I wouldn't do that, if I were you." It is Janet making one last try.

I dial the number. Gloria answers, someone I have known for years. I request that my chart be set aside for me. "I'll be there this afternoon," I tell her.

"No problem," says Gloria. But three hours later she calls to say that my chart has been misplaced. It is nowhere to be found . . . it hadn't ever come down from the ward . . . they are turning the place upside down . . . she will phone again as soon as they find it.

"Just as well," says Janet. "Remember Lot's wife? Best not to look back."

Truth to tell, I feel some relief along with my exasperation. Perhaps I shouldn't read it after all? Four weeks later, the chart will still not have been found.

July 18: My brother Billy arrives.

"Did they finally ever figure out what you had?"

"Dutch elm disease."

"For goodness' sake, I thought only plants . . ."

"Not at all. I caught it from an infected tree. I was taking a nap under it."

He stands to leave. "I guess Jesus didn't want you for a sunbeam yet." All at once, the valves of my brother's heart swing open and I can see what flutters inside—love.

July 24: At ten o'clock at night the phone rings. I have been asleep for two hours. It is Gordon, my doctor.

"Just calling to see how you are."

"It's the dead of night. *Non sum qualis eram*."

"What's that?"

"Latin for I am not what I used to be. What do you want?"

"Great doctor-patient relationship we have going here. I am just now reading one of your books. I don't usually cry but you . . ."

"Well, you made me cry plenty. It's your turn."

"Well, how are you? It's my duty to ask."

"I'm not sure. I'd have to read my chart to find out, and they can't find it." I tell him about the cough, how it keeps me awake.

"You back to writing yet?"

"No."

"Why not?"

"The synaptic spark, it's gone. All that prolonged hypoxia to the brain."

"Oh, come on! Where'd you get all that about prolonged hypoxia? You're not getting depressed, are you? Still having nightmares? Been back to the Nile delta lately?"

"I'm tired. I'm lightheaded. I can't keep my thoughts straight."

"Go back to sleep."

I lie back, thinking of Patrick. How, dipping a plastic urinal, he poured water over my head, then palmed the cake of soap and worked it into a lather.

"When I get t'rough wit' ye . . ." The Irishman's face, ruddy and shining from the humidity . . . It is months later and still my thoughts return to it as to a sacrament.

July 28: I am like that sultan in the Turkish fairy tale who was told by a dervish to stick his head in a pail of water. The sultan did so and when he removed it, he learned that he had aged thirty years, most of which he had spent in captivity. He learned too that he had fathered children and grandchildren.

I have the distinct sensation that every afternoon

grass is growing inside my head. Three weeks and two days! People say: "In three weeks . . ." or "Three weeks ago . . ." without thinking what can happen in the space of three weeks. And two days. For some, three weeks is the gist, the core of a lifetime, on either side of which the years stretch out as if they were adjuncts to that molten, vivid three weeks. And two days.

August 1: A phone call to the record room confirms that the chart is still lost. Fine. In the absence of any record of my illness, I shall write it myself. Invent it out of whole cloth. It is what a writer can do that a doctor cannot.

Already the story begins to unfold in my mind: there is the suddenness of onset, the absence of premonitory signs or symptoms. Like John Donne, one minute I was well, and sick the next. There is the daily shrinkage of the flesh around the ever more prominent skeleton, the wild swings in temperature; there is the peripheral vascular collapse with falling blood pressure, impalpable pulse, persistent cyanosis. The X-ray shows a dense white blizzard of pneumonia throughout both lungs.

What's this! What's this! The patient is swollen with fluid from excessive hydration. How could they have done that? The liver-function tests are abnormal. Microscopic casts have appeared in the urine. And, in the corridor just outside the doorway but within earshot, are the doctors pulling at their beards, using the professional plural: "Should we add erythromycin? Steroids? What about a tracheotomy?" It is a very iliad of woes.

It shouldn't be too hard to write. Hadn't I made thousands of entries in the charts of thousands of my own patients? I know just the proper tone of voice to use—austere, pragmatic, economical. For some days, I have been jotting down snatches, not as a story, mind you, only a detail here and there as it comes back to me, small things stored in the lumber room of the mind. Sometimes, though, what comes back is so fierce as to abolish the time interval between the event and my recollection of it, so that it recurs in all its original fury. Then I fidget in the lawn chair and start to cough. At last I must reach for my cane and go into the house.

August 15: In the kitchen at 5 A.M. Make coffee. Cast a few grains of rice into the spoon drawer. Moments later comes the *tack-tack-tack* of tiny claws, or is it the clicking of microscopic teeth to let me know that the offering has been accepted? One must take care of one's little household gods. Also, I keep the neighbor's cats out of the house. All this I do, not in appeasement, but out of a Franciscan respect for beasts and insects. Not long ago I too was a creature on the edge of extinction, some featherless, beakless bird dependent upon the sacrifices of others. Besides, this mouse has been in the spoon drawer for months. He has many more ancestors than I.

Doubtless, he feels himself more estimable than I by far.

Again and again I read over the notes I have made. And each time with increasing dissatisfaction. As a hospital record, it is adequate, I suppose. But I no longer write those. I write stories. And as a story, it lacks acceleration, crescendo, suspense and subtlety, irony, humor, the grotesque, all of the writerly stunts I have used so many times before. Most glaring is the absence of that single critical event that would raise the chronicle above the ordinary, a climax. What, I wonder, can it be that would shatter the sophistication of the hospital, the complacence of the doctors? Something, I think, supernatural, that cannot be explained in accordance with the laws of nature.

I do not know precisely when the idea occurred to me that only death and resurrection would suffice. But dying? you say. It's a bit extreme. Why tempt fate? And resurrections are tricky. Have you ever known one to come off without a hitch? Never mind. A writer will go to any lengths to captivate and entertain his readers. And I am no better than I should be. So it is decided that, after twenty-three days in the intensive care unit, I died. A nice touch, that twenty-three, like the psalm of that number: *Yea, though I walk through the valley of the shadow of death . . .*

Best, I think, to tell it with a minimum of ornamentation. No metaphors, similes, imagery. Just words of one syllable, a monochrome. That should balance whatever element of the spectacular may be inherent in the event. Only, at the instant of resurrection, there will be that silent stillness that fell upon the earth when Jesus Christ was born. Followed by a soft drumming on the roof. Had it begun to rain? Or was it the return of the heartbeat? And a lucidity that was almost unbearable filling the mind. In a moment, one's head would burst open . . .

Where to turn for a precedent? The account in the gospel of the raising of Lazarus is skimpy, to say the least. To sum up: Lazarus was a close friend of Jesus. It came to pass that Lazarus fell ill and died and was buried in his tomb. But the sisters of Lazarus, Martha and Mary, came weeping to Christ and asked why he had not saved their brother. Either Jesus was moved or else it was time for another miracle. He resurrected Lazarus, who had been dead for four days. I see the man now as Rembrandt did—sitting up in the darkness of his tomb, peeling off his cerements, a look of wonder on his pallid face.

Unlike Lazarus, I'll stay dead for only ten minutes. Considering the unusually warm weather last April, delicacy alone forbids a longer death. Besides, ten minutes is quite enough to experience whatever it is that lies on the yonder side of the grave, what the gullible call the hereafter. Already, I admit to no small pleasure at the prospect of former colleagues sheepishly probing for news of what and whom I encountered on the other side.

"How did it happen?" they'll ask. "What was it like?"

"It was like this: there was nothing; I was not. And then I was."

"That's all?"

"Yes, that's all."

"No, no! What was it like?"

"What was *what* like?"

"You know . . . dying, then . . . coming back?"

"Oh, that. It's like a dream in which you think, *I've already dreamt that.*"

"And the coming back part?"

"Wait a minute . . . I have to think . . . it's a cold, tingling green."

"An immersion then?"

"Not really. More like a hard slap."

"Oh."

Day by day I drift deeper into misty eccentricity. One day I may simply vanish therein. Just today Janet came into my study.

"What are you writing down there all day?"

"The chronicle of my illness."

"How is it going?"

"In a word, *marvelously.*"

"Really? Read me what you just wrote."

"At precisely that moment over the loudspeaker came the loud crowing of a rooster. After the monotonous calling out of names of doctors and phone extensions, the effect was stunning. Again and again:

Cock-a-doodle-doo! At which, wherever in the vast hospital they were—morgue, kitchen, laundry, operating theater, emergency suite, nursery—the faithful fell to their knees, aves foaming from their lips. For it is well known that the rooster is the bird of resurrection."

"That's what you just wrote?"

"Yes. What do you think?"

"You're kidding." Silence. "Come on, say you're kidding."

To be congenial, then: "I'm kidding."

September 10: The chart is written. Down to the last hallelujah. And perhaps it is not all a mere conceit, a figment of the imagination. Perhaps it is truer than had it been woven from the facts. The facts are not always where the truth lies. Ask the great historians, for whom the facts are there to be interpreted anew by each generation of scholars. Facts have a way of changing from time to time. The truth lies beneath the surface of the facts. What! you say. In coma and he can see and hear and perceive all of that? Why not? Noah saw the world most clearly during the forty days that he was shut up inside the ark, despite the utter darkness that reigned.

The more I think about it, the more real my death and resurrection become. There are whole afternoons when I have no doubt that it happened. About the next world? The truth? I don't remember a darn thing about it. Now and then, sitting in this garden, I have the faint recollection of a finger placed across my lips, shushing me. And of a voice (was it a voice?) uttering the words THOU SHALT NOT. There is a vague familiarity about it, as though I had received the same pressure on my mouth once before, long ago. So! It was as my mother said then:

"What's this groove?" I asked her. I pointed from my nose to my lip.

"Ask your father."

"It's called the philtrum," he said. "It's where the two halves of your face join before you are born, only there is that little depression left."

"No," said Mother with all the authority of the one who had carried me in that red darkness between her hips. "It is the finger of the shushing angel, whose job it is to warn the newborn babies not to reveal the secrets of life before birth." It was the same angel on duty for resurrections.

October 15: I have exchanged the broad-brimmed straw hat for a beret. Janet is pruning and mulching instead of planting and hoeing. I no longer cough. Every morning with my loyal cane I walk the eight blocks to the Yale library, then back home every afternoon. I have taken to pecking at the bones of an old short story, trying to prod it to its feet. There is a phone call from the hospital. It is Gloria from the records room.

"Good news!" she says. "We've found your chart. I've put it aside for you—all three volumes."

"Oh good. Well . . . yes," I tell her. "I'll come around before long." But of course I won't. It is much too late. I've already written my chart, and no mere hospital record could match it for pathos and narrative drive. Besides, I've turned my back on all of that. I'm going to spend the rest of the autumn groping my way back to my work, hoping to sprout some new green shoots from the ends of lopped branches, which so far have produced only a gray, bronchial prose. About that death and resurrection? Well, art is a means of acquiring experiences that one never had. Let's leave it at that.

December 1: There is more than a suggestion of winter in the air, especially in the early mornings. Thinking about my Legionnaires' disease has grown tiresome. One final observation has to do with my fingernails. Only days ago, I noticed at some two-thirds of the distance between each cuticle and the tip of the finger a fine, distinct transverse dent. Now, considering that fingernail grows at an average rate of one millimeter per week, and considering that the length of the nail proximal to the crease measures two centimeters, it cannot fail to occur to even the least suggestible that these lines were at the very nail bed itself some twenty weeks ago. That would be April, sometime during my comatose residency in the intensive care unit. What are these transverse creases if not the manifestation of some cataclysmic event that took place at that time? Rather like the geological evidence of a prehistoric earthquake or an interplanetary collision.

It takes no great leap of the imagination (mine, at least) to connect these lines with the death and resurrection that I had thought to be the product of a writer's fancy. These little marks on my fingernails give witness that for the duration of that "death," the fingernails ceased to grow and only resumed growing after the resurrection. It is further evidence, if any were needed, that life imitates art, and not the other way around. Nor has any doctor to whom I have shown these markings come up with a better hypothesis, least of all my own doctor, to whose office I raced with the electrifying evidence.

"Oh those," said Gordon, yawning behind a fist. "Beau's lines. We see them after major medical disorders—a coronary, severe pneumonia." As if familiarity could diminish the miraculous.

"So you have seen them before?" I respond. "But can you explain why they occur?"

"No, I am afraid we cannot."

"Well then," I replied and stepped out of his examining room and back into my life.

• • •